# A LOOK INTO MYASTHENIA GRAVIS

Edited by **Joseph A. Pruitt**

**A Look into Myasthenia Gravis**
Edited by Joseph A. Pruitt

**Published by InTech**

Janeza Trdine 9, 51000 Rijeka, Croatia



**Publishing Process Manager** Oliver Kurelic

**Technical Editor** Teodora Smiljanic

**Cover Designer** InTech Design Team

Additional hard copies can be obtained from orders@intechopen.com

A Look into Myasthenia Gravis, Edited by Joseph A. Pruitt
p. cm.
ISBN 978-953-307-821-2

For EU product safety concerns:
IN TECH d.o.o., Prolaz Marije Krucifikse Kozulić 3, 51000 Rijeka, Croatia,
info@intechopen.com or visit our website at intechopen.com.

# Meet the editor

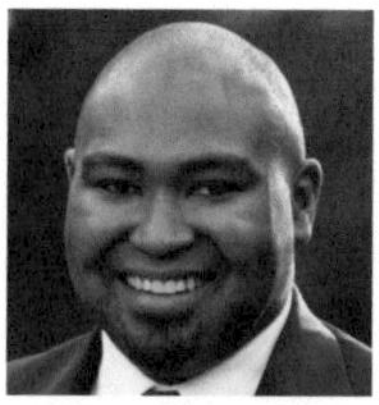

Dr Joseph A. Pruitt, OD, MBA, FAAO, received his Bachelor of Science degree in Biology from California State Polytechnic University, his Doctor of Optometry degree from the Illinois College of Optometry, and his Master of Business Administration degree from H. Wayne Huizenga School of Business and Entrepreneurship at Nova Southeastern University. Dr Pruitt completed a residency in Geriatric/Primary Care Optometry at the West Los Angeles Veteran Affairs Healthcare Center, and is Board Certified by the American Board of Certification in Medical Optometry. In addition to that, he is a Fellow of the American Academy of Optometry. Dr Pruitt resides and practices in the United States.

# Contents

# Preface

This publication is the result of the joining of forces, so to speak, of a diverse group of professionals in an effort to depict the many manifestations of myasthenia gravis. Although, in the grand scheme of things, only a few manifestations are covered in this text, the far-reaching effect of this disease is not lost. From the surgical treatment of the disease's complications to the common findings of a routine eye examination, this text explores this disease's impact in a variety of outlets within healthcare. We hope you find this text interesting, but most importantly informative. Enjoy.

**Joseph A. Pruitt**
Minneapolis Veterans Affairs Medical Center,
Minneapolis, Minnesota,
University of Missouri-Saint Louis College of Optometry,
Saint Louis, Missouri
USA

# Part 1

## Clinical Presentations

# 1

# Myasthenia Gravis with Anti-MuSK Antibodies: Clinical Features and Histopathological Changes

Corrado Angelini[1,2], Sara Martignago[1], Michela Biscigli[1] and Elisa Albertini[1]
[1]*Department of Neurosciences, University of Padova, Padova*
[2]*IRCCS San Camillo; Venezia*
*Italy*

## 1. Introduction

Myasthenia gravis (MG) is a neuromuscular autoimmune disorder caused by binding of autoantibodies to molecules involved in neuromuscular transmission: acetylcholine receptor (AChR) and muscle specific tyrosine kinase (MuSK). It is characterized by a fluctuant weakness.

The most typical feature is a painless, variable weakness of skeletal muscles that worsens with exercise and improves with rest. It may involve different muscles and frequently the presenting symptoms are ptosis and/or diplopia due to the involvement of extraocular muscles. MG diagnosis is based on a detailed clinical history, on pharmacological test and on the measurement of antibodies against the Acetylcholine receptor (AchR-Ab). Some MG patients do not have detectable AChR-Ab and have been defined as "seronegative" (SNMG) (Vincent 2004). A high proportion of these patients have purely ocular symptoms (ocular MG). Seronegative generalized myasthenia is proving to be heterogeneous on clinical, immunological and histopathological features. A variable proportion of SNMG patients has antibodies against MuSK. These antibodies are directed against the extracellular domain of MuSK and inhibit the agrin-induced AChR clustering in muscle myotubes. Although the role of these antibodies in causing myasthenic symptoms in vivo is not still clear, MuSK antibodies appear to define a group of patients.

## 2. Pathophysiology

The neuromuscular junction (NMJ) is the communication between nerve and muscle where the electrical nerve impulse is translated into an electrical stimulation to initiate muscle contraction [1]. Acetylcholine (ACh) acts as the chemical messenger between the nerve fibre and the postsynaptic muscle membrane. ACh is released into the synaptic cleft on nerve depolarization and rapidly diffuses to bind to ACh receptors (AChRs). AChRs can be either nicotinic or muscarinic. The nicotinic AChR is a multimeric protein comprised in adults of two $\alpha$ subunits and one each of $\beta$, $\delta$, and $\varepsilon$ subunits. The nicotinic AChR is a multimeric protein made of two $\alpha$ subunits, which in turn are made of $\beta$, $\delta$, and $\varepsilon$ subunits. Each $\alpha$

subunit has a binding site for ACh. Muscle-specific tyrosine kinase (MuSK) is an AChR-associated protein involved in clustering of AChR during synapse formation and is expressed in the mature NMJ [2].

Autoimmune disorders result from the loss of tolerance to self-antigens. In the case of myasthenia gravis (MG), an autoimmune disorder characterized by clinical fatigable weakness, the body raises an autoimmune attack on its own muscle endplate, initiated by antibody binding to AChR or, less frequently, to MuSK, resulting in abnormal neuromuscular transmission and muscle weakness.

Approximately 80% of patients have detectable serum antibodies against AChR that reduce AChR number and impair their function at the neuromuscular endplate. About 15-30% of MG patients do not have detectable AChRAb and are defined as *seronegative*. These patients may have purely ocular symptoms but a small proportion has generalized weakness. About half of seronegative MG cases has antibodies against a muscle-specific tyrosine-kinase protein (MuSK-Ab). The role of MuSK-Ab in the pathogenesis of MG is still unclear. These antibodies probably impair neuromuscular transmission, as MuSK protein plays a critical role in postsynaptic differentiation and in AChR gene expression [3]. MuSK is a transmembrane polypeptide selectively expressed in skeletal muscle. It is part of the agrin-receptor, an essential protein in building the neuromuscular synapses. Experimental data show that agrin-induced activation of MuSK by tyrosine phosphorylation results in aggregation and expression of specific muscle proteins, AChR included, and in AChR phosphorylation [4]. Anti-MuSK serum antibodies may bind the external domain and reduce the agrin-induced expression of AChR in myotubes in vitro [5]· Selcen et al. Demonstrated in a single patient on intercostal muscle biopsy, that MuSK-Ab do not cause a reduction of MuSK or AChR in neuromuscular plate [6], but its presence in the neuromuscular junction causes a 20% decrease of AChR-clusters and a decrease of agrin-induced AChR-clusters according to study in all patients [7]. MuSK-Ab also do not cause internalization of AChR, as demonstrated in AChR-Ab MG [7].

The thymus is a critical organ for T-cell education and elimination of auto-reactive T-cells, and plays a major role in MG. Thymic abnormalities are frequently present in MG, including hyperplasia in about 65% of cases and thymoma in 10%. The expression of AChR by myoid cells in the thymus plus the inflammatory environment within the MG thymus, contribute to the induction and maintenance of the anti-AChR autoimmune response [8].

## 3. Epidemiology

MG used to be considered a rare disease, however incidence and prevalence rates have increased over time, partly as a result of increased of diagnosis, and results of prolonged survival with the disease for new improvement protocol of patients [9]. the current incidence rates range from 9–21 per million population, with prevalence rates of 50–125 cases per million population worldwide.

The onset and incidence of MG is influenced by age and gender and MG was first thought to be a condition of the young female and old male. Epidemiological data show that women are most frequently affected than men; age at onset in MG patients with MuSK-Ab occurs predominantly before 40 years, at a younger age than MG cases with AChR-Ab [9]. Women are frequently more affected than men [10; 11]. Recent reports indicate that MG may be under-diagnosed in the elderly [12].

## 4. Clinical features

Patients with MG present weakness in specific muscle groups. The main feature is a fluctuant variable weakness of skeletal muscles that worsens with exercise and improves with rest. The onset in about the 65% of patients is characterised by ocular symptoms, such as ptosis and diplopia, the remaining 25% of patients shows bulbar weakness, resulting in slurred or nasal speech, voice alterations or difficulty in chewing or swallowing. Limb weakness is a less common initial complaint [13; 14]. The degree of weakness may vary during the day, but, generally it worsens with exercises and improve with rest.

The progression of muscle weakness in MG usually occurs in a craniocaudal direction, beginning with ocular, facial, lower bulbar muscles, and progressing to torso and limb muscle involvement. Maximal weakness occurs within the first year following the onset of the disease in approximately two-thirds of the cases [15; 16]. Up to 50% of patients who presents ocular MG will progress to generalized MG within 6 months, rising up to 80% within 2 years [14].

However, in around 10–40% of cases, muscle weakness remains restricted to the ocular muscles. [13]

MG with anti-MuSK-Ab has a different phenotype from the remaining seronegative MG; in most of the cases symptoms at onset includes nasal voice, weakness of facial and limb muscles and respiratory muscles [17; 16]. Patients can show a severe predominantly facio-bulbar weakness with dyspnea and nasal speech; dysphagia sometimes is so severe that it leads to an important weight loss. In some cases, only ocular muscles can be affected [18]. A significant association between bulbar/facial muscles weakness and muscular atrophy has been described in MuSK-positive patients [7], this could justify the selective and typical bulbar involvement.

MG remains a challenging disease to diagnose due to its fluctuating character and to the similarity of symptoms to those of other disorders; the mean time to diagnosis is often over 1 year [13; 14]. Seronegative MG with anti-MuSK antibodies still remains a diagnostic challenge, because of its fluctuating character and the similarity of symptoms to with other disorders. Mean time to diagnosis is often over 1 year [13; 14]. The diagnostic value of neostigmine or edrophonium test and repetitive stimulation is low [15], while single fibre EMG has very high sensitivity.

MG with MuSK-Ab is responsive to standard therapy, but needs higher drug dosages than MG AChR-Ab positive [19], MuSK-positive patients frequently develop hypersensitivity to anticholinesterase drugs [15]. Instead, seronegative MG without MuSK-Ab seems to have a similar or less severe clinical course than seropositive ones and a similar response to pharmacological treatment [20].

## 5. Treatment

The treatment of MG includes both a surgical and a therapeutic approach.

**Thymectomy** is currently performed in patients with thymoma (usually by median sternotomy) and in generalized AChR-positive MG (cervicotomy, VATS, VATET), where it appears to increase the rate of remission. In MuSK-positive MG, thymectomy is generally thought to be of less value and the question of whether it has a role in the disease treatment is controversial. This opinion is based on clinical reports and morphological studies. These studies [17, 19], even if performed in small patient series and presenting potential confounding factors such as the effect of immunosuppressive treatment and the inclusion of patients with different disease severity and duration, have altogether failed to show a better outcome in thymectomised than in unthymectomised MuSK-positive patients, both in terms of remission rate and need for immunosuppressive therapy.

**Drugs:** Symptomatic drugs, such as anticholinesterase, are generally well tolerated and represent the first-line treatment in most patients, they can improve muscle strength in a minority of cases [21]. Immunosuppressive therapy is indicated for patients with symptoms not controlled with acetyl-cholinesterase inhibitors. Different drugs have been used alone or in combination: corticosteroids, azathioprine, cyclosporine, cyclophosphamide, mycophenolate mofetil, tacrolimus, and rituximab [21] (Table I). In the AChR-positive disease, immunosuppressive therapy is highly effective. Short-term treatments, such as plasma-exchange (PE) and intravenous immunoglobulin (IVIG), are used to treat patients with severe, rapidly progressing disease. The response to therapy in MuSK-positive MG patients seems to be different from that in AChR-Ab positive. In MuSK-positive MG the response to anchtiolinesterase is generally unsatisfactory. A general impression is that MuSK MG patients fare worse than AChR-Ab-positive patients [22]. This impression is based on the remission rate. When comparing therapeutic results in MuSK-MG and AChR-MG in a meta-analysis, Evoli et al.[17] found a significant difference in remission rates: 10%–35% in MuSK-MG versus 24%–58% in AChR-MG. Because of the disease severity and the poor response to acetyl-cholinesterase inhibitors, the majority of MuSK-positive patients require immunosuppressive therapy [22].

## 6. Histopathological changes in muscles and thymus

Thymus pathology in MuSK-positive patients is not so far available because of the relatively minor incidence of this subgroup in the population of myasthenic patients. MG is initiated within the thymus by immunogenic presentation of locally produced nicotinic acetylcholine receptor (AChR) to potentially autoimmune T cells [23]. Because the thymus is the central organ for immunological self-tolerance, it is reasonable to suspect that thymic abnormalities cause the breakdown in tolerance that causes an immune-mediated attack on AChR in myasthenia gravis. The thymus contains myoid cells that express the AChR antigen, antigen presenting cells, and immunocompetent T-cells. Thymus tissue from patients with myasthenia gravis produces AChR antibodies when implanted into immunodeficient mice. However, in AChR-negative/MuSK-positive MG, the thymus does not appear to play such an important role in the pathogenesis as it is thought to play in non- thymoma seropositive MG [24].

Pathological studies often demonstrate thymic hyperplasia in AChR-Ab positive and in AChR-ab negative/MuSK-negative patients. In contrast, in the thymuses from MuSK-positive patients, lymphoid follicles with germinal centres are not found and the perivascular space harbors amounts of lymphoid cells are significantly less than in the

| Pt. Sex | Age at onset | Age at last follow up | Years of disease | MGFA score at onset | Thymectomy | Muscle biopsy | Therapy * | | | | MGFA score at last follow up ^ |
|---|---|---|---|---|---|---|---|---|---|---|---|
| | | | | | | | ACH | STER | IM | PE/IVIG | |
| **1 F** | 43 | 49 | 6 | II a | Robotic Thymic atrophy | + | X | X | X | X | II a |
| **2 M** | 27 | 45 | 17 | III b | | + | X | X | X | X | II b |
| **3 F** | 34 | 39 | 5 | IV b | Rodotic Hyperlplasia | + | X | X | X | X | II b |
| **4 F** | 24 | 30 | 6 | II a | | | X | X | | | AS |
| **5 F** | 50 | 50 | 1 | II b | Sternothomy Hyperplasia | + | X | X | X | X | III b |
| **6 F** | 22 | 44 | 21 | III b | | + | X | X | X | X | II b |
| **7 F** | 41 | 46 | 5 | IV b | VATET Hyperplasia | + | X | X | X | X | II b |
| **8F** | 45 | 53 | 8 | II b | | + | X | X | X | X | II b |
| **9 F** | 45 | 46 | 2 | III b | | | X | X | | X | AS |

* ACH. anticholineterases; STER. Steroid; IM. Immunosoppressive drugs; PE. Plasma exchange
^ AS asintomatic

Table I. Clinical characteristics and therapy efficacy in MuSK-positive MG

AChR-Ab patients. Thymus changes in these cases resemble those in normal aging [25]. Thymectomy often results in clinical improvement in AChR-Ab positive patients, suggesting a role for the thymus in the initiation or propagation of the autoimmune attack on the myocyte. The role of thymectomy in MuSK-positive MG remains uncertain. Recent studies reported no reduction in immunosuppressive therapy or reduction in MuSK antibody titles following thymectomy, and no difference in clinical status between MuSK MG patients with or without thymectomy [17].

**Diagnosis procedure in Myastenia gravis and muscle biopsy morphology**

The diagnosis of MG is based on clinical, laboratory and instrumental procedures; muscles biopsy is performed only to exclude alternative diagnosis therefore the number of muscle biopsies available is limited. Muscle biopsy of intercostal muscles in mostly used in congenital myasthenia. The biopsied muscles are usually the limb muscles (quadriceps, deltoid) thus the pathology could be different in bulbar muscles that can't be examined.

The muscle biopsies of AChR-Ab positive patients shows focal and usually non-specific changes. They include atrophy of type 2 fibers, and sometimes atrophy of type 1 fibers, and rarely the presence of small angulated fibers and fiber type grouping, suggestive of denervation [26]. Ultrastrucural images of ednplate show the presence of reduced folds of the junction, and debris from them accumulates between the nerve and the muscle membrane. Complement and immune complexes can be demonstrated on the post-synaptic membrane, as well as the binding of autoantibodies in the serum from affected patients to neuromuscular junction has been observed. In the past no study was done to study electron microscopy or histopathology of MuSK positive biopsies. In our study [27], we analysed muscle biopsy of 13 myasthenic patients (8 women and 5 men), whose diagnosis was based on standard criteria. Seven patients were positive for AChR-Ab (serum AChRAb > 0.25 nmol/l) and six positive for MuSK-Ab and negative for AChR-Ab. Our findings reveal that MG associated with antibodies against MuSK and MG associated to AChR-Ab show different histopathological features. Atrophy factor in skeletal muscle biopsies is higher for both type I and type II fibers in AChR-Ab positive cases: this feature agrees with the observation that the disease affects more severely the limb than the bulbar muscles (Figure 1). Atrophy of type II fibers might be explained by a reduced muscle strength and disuse atrophy in both groups of patients. Skeletal muscle fibres of MuSK-positive cases are relatively preserved by atrophy, and this could be due either to a focal action of MuSK antibodies or to the fact that bulbar muscles are the onlyone partially susceptible to MuSK antibodies. In this study we observed prominent signs of mitochondrial involvement, such as COX-negative fibers or mitochondrial aggregates and myofibrillar disarray, in MuSK-positive patients, indicating that mitochondrial function could have a role in this disease (Figure 2). The presence of several COX negative fibers in patients under 40 years can be regarded as abnormal, aince SOX.fibres are not usually seen until after 50 years. In contrast, AChR-Ab positive showed only mild and unspecific myopathic changes, but often muscle fibre atrophy and few aggregates of normally shaped mitochondria were observed.

The ultrastructured study of biopsy from MuSK-positive patients [27] confirmed the pattern of severe myopathic changes, such as swollen mithochondria, myofibrillar loss, and sarcoplasmic reticulum lipid vesicles associated with enlarged mithocondria with electronlucent matrix and fragmented cristae [28]. Mitochondria are aggregated both in the subsarcolemmal and intermyofibrillar areas (Figure 3), adjacent to normal mitochondria.

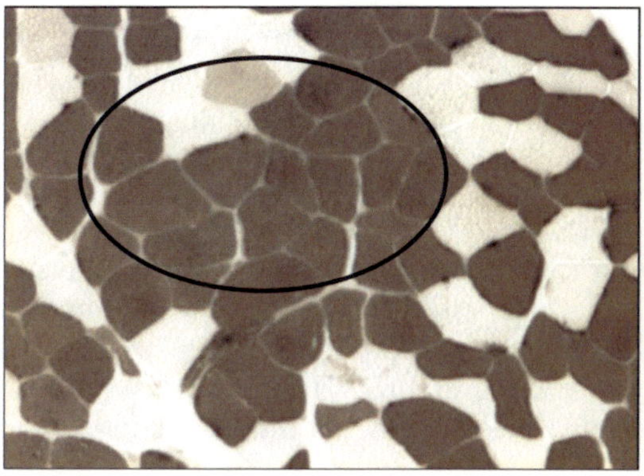

Fig. 1. Light microscopy. Acid ATP-ase stain shows type I fibre grouping in one AChR-Ab patient

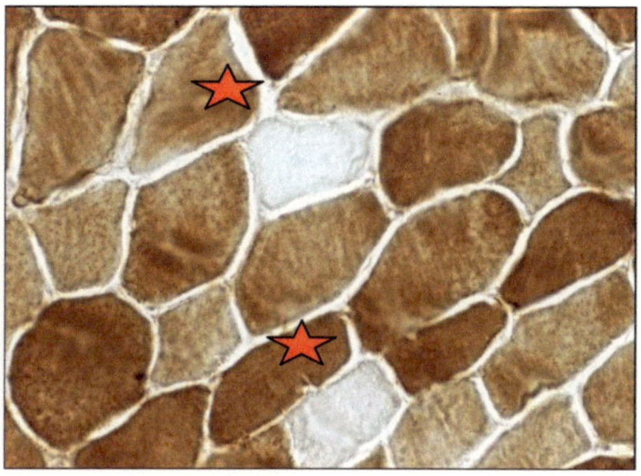

Fig. 2. COX stain shows 2 COX-negative fibers (star) in one AChR-Ab patient.

Ultrastructural studies show also that MuSK-positive cause a 20% decrease of AChR number on the surface of the postsynaptic membrane, clusters of AChR in MuSK-positive patients appear larger than in AChR-Ab positive cases, and this could be due to cluster dispersion induced by MuSK antibodies (Figure 4). These antibodies cause a decrease of AChR agrin-induced expression [2, 4]. The presence of fiber type grouping in many AChR+ patients might be explained by blockage of AChR receptor binding that causes the internalization and degradation of AChR and consequently a denervation of affected muscle [29]. Fiber type grouping in cases with anti-MuSK-Ab is less frequently observed. In a recent study of Rostedt Punga *et al.* [30] deltoid muscle of 10 MuSK+ and 40 AChR+ patients were compared. They analized mtDNA in the cases that presented histological mitochondrial

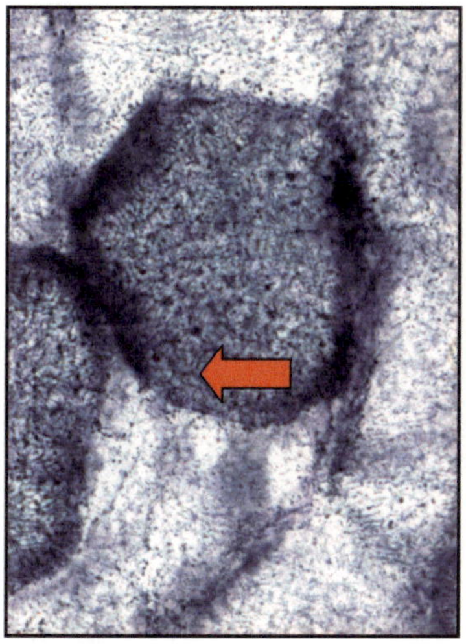

Fig. 3. NADH-TR stain. Subsarcolemmal mitochondrial rims in one MuSK-positive patient

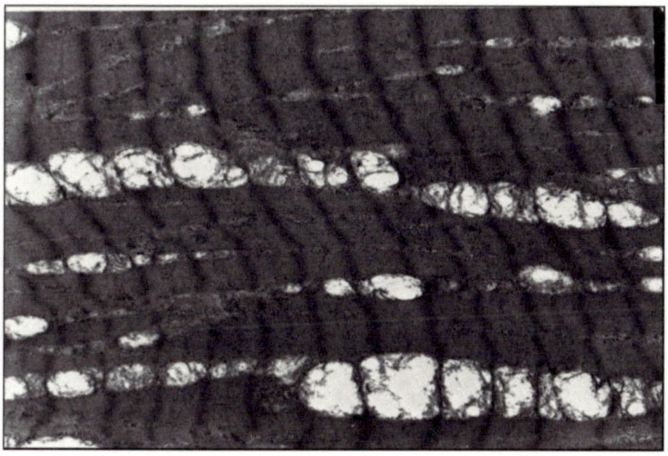

Fig. 4. Swelling of mitochondria and cristae disruption in MuSK-positive. Dense mitochondria were disposed perpendicular to the sarcomeres

abnormalities at muscle specimens, and they found frequent deletions in mtDNA, supporting the morphological date.

In conclusion, atrophy could bedue to a functional denervation in AChR-Ab positive patients while, in MuSK-positive patients, there are mild myopathic changes with prominent mitochondrial abnormalities.

Clinical aspects, electrophysiological tests, immunological presentation, thymus pathology and the therapeutic response implicate that MG MuSK-positive is a specific subgroup of seronegative MG, and has to be analised as a peculiar muscle pathology. Treatment and diagnosis, as well as prognosis and surgical approach is different in MG with MuSK-Ab. The clinician should be alerted of this different bfeatures and have a different approach to this tipe of myasthenia gravis.

## 7. Anti-MuSK patients in clinical practice

In our Neuromuscular Centre Database we collected 279 MG patients: 171 female and 108 male. AChR-Ab were positive in 143 patients positive (51%). Among the 97 seronegative patients (35%) only 46 (16%) presented a generalized MG: MuSK-Ab were positive in 9 of them (19%).

Diagnosis was based on standard criteria [13,31], including symptoms of fluctuating muscle fatigue, supported by an electromyographic pattern (repetitive nerve stimulation). Patients were periodically examined at the Neuromuscular Diseases Centre, University of Padova. MG classification had been performed according to the Myasthenia Gravis Foundation of America. MGFA class I includes only ocular onset; class II includes mild generalized onset; class III includes moderate generalized onset; class IV includes severe generalized fatigue; class V patients need intubation. For classes II–IV, a further classification in subclass 'a' indicates prevalent limb muscle involvement, while subclass 'b' includes patients with predominant bulbar muscle involvement. Muscle strength was determined using MRC score (Medical Research Council) of every biopsied muscle at time of diagnosis. MRC score: 5 - normal force, 4 - movement against gravity and resistance, 3 - movement just against gravity, 2 - movement is possible just in absence of gravity, 1 - muscle contraction is visible but no movement is seen and 0 - no contraction is visible. Plus and minus indicates an intermediate degree of muscle strength. The clinical data collected included: age at onset, sex, therapy assessment and muscle strength conditions at the time of diagnosis.

The MuSK-positive patient were 8 females and one male with a mean age at onset of 47 ± 19.7 (Table I). At onset 2 of them presented generalized symptoms and were both in II-a MGFA score class; 7 (78%) presented bulbar symptoms: 2 were in class II-b, 3 in class III-b and 2 in class IV-b of MGFA score. Four (44%) were thymectomised: one had a thymic atrophy and 3 (75%) thymic hyperplasia.

Biopsy was done in seven patients at the time of MG diagnosis. Histopathological investigations were performed blind to the patient's clinical status. Muscle biopsies of patients were collected after informed consent; all procedures were conducted after obtaining the approval from the University Review Board.

At the last follow-up visit, after a mean duration of disease of 10 years, six patients were improved: two patients were asymptomatic, four were in class II-b. Two patients were unchanged and only one got worse. Corticosteroids associated with anticholinesterases were sufficient only in one patient; 8 (89%) needed an additional treatment with immunosuppressive drug: four used azathioprine and had to change therapy for unsatisfactory response to the first-one: three pass to cyclosporine and one to mycophenolate mofetil. One patient used cyclosporine since MG onset. Eight patients (89%) were treated with IVIG and had a clinical improvement. PE was used in three patients, with a minor response.

| Agent (trade names) | Initial dose | Maintenance dose | Onset of action |
|---|---|---|---|
| **Prednisone** | 15-20mg q.d., Increasing by 5-10mg q2-3 days | 1.5 mg/kg/day, followed by slow alternate day taper (taper by 5-10mg a month) | 2-4 weeks |
| **Azathioprine** | 50mg q.d. * | Increase by 50mg increments q 2-4 weeks to target of 2-3 mg/kg | 2-10 months for initial response, up to 24 months for peak |
| **Cyclosporin** | 100mg b.i.d. ^ | Increase slowly as needed to 3-6 mg/kg on b.i.d. schedule | 1-3 months |
| **Mycophenolate** | 500mg b.i.d. | 1000-1500mg b.i.d. | 2-12 months |
| **Cyclophosphamide** | 3-5 mg/kg/day, can be preceded by intravenous pulse | 2-3 mg/kg a day | 2-6 months |
| **Tacrolimus/FK-506** | 3-5 mg/day or 0.1 mg/kg/day | Increase up to 5-7mg a day following dosage of plasmatic levels | 1-3 months |
| **Rituximab** | 375 mg/m2 IV every 1-2 weeks for 4 weeks | None or 375 mg/m2 every 4-10 weeks for a few months | 1-3 months |
| **Etanercept** | 25mg s.c. ° twice weekly | 25mg s.c. twice weekly | 2- months |

^ b.i.d., twice daily;
* q.d., daily;
° s.c., subcutaneous

Table II. Commonly used immunosuppressant agents for myasthenia gravis

## 8. Case Report

A 36 years-old woman presented 2 years history of progressive dyspnea and fatigue. She complained of diffuse weakness. She had no complaint for pain or cramps but noticed an increased difficulty in climbing stairs. She had a nasal speech, but denied diplopia and ptosis. She had lost 40 kg for a progressive and severe difficulty in swallowing solid food.

Past medical history was positive only for a hiatus hernia and esophageal gastrointestinal reflux. EMG, brain MRI and mediastinial CT gave normal results. Pneumological evaluation showed a high breathways obstructive pattern.

Examination revealed normal vital signs: her gait was slow; strength testing revealed mild weakness in triceps (4+/5), deltoid and brachioradialis (4/5), gastrocnemius (5-/5) and in orbicularis oculi et oris. Extensive auto-immunity battery examination gave normal results, except for the research of anti-MuSK antibodies, that were positive. Pneumological evaluation showed a slight restrictive pattern.

Logopedic evaluation documented dysphonia and slowed deglutition. There was a depressive psychological profile. Electrodiagnostic studies with repetitive nerve stimulation were normal. Muscle biopsy revealed atrophy of muscle fibers, minicores and mitocondrial alterations. Treatment with trazodone and tocopherol was started. Despite this treatment, her condition worsened because of persistent dysphagia and rhinolalia; respiratory insufficiency became so severe that she needed a mechanical assisted ventilation during the night. IVIg and cyclosporine reversed her condition and brought a permanent improvement.

The final diagnosis was: MuSK-positive myasthenia with anorexia and ventilatory insufficiency.

This study is supported by Eurobiobank, TREAT-NMD, Telethon GUP 07001 and Grant from Italian Ministry of Education. We thank also myasthenia gravis patients that collaborated to this study.

## 9. References

[1] Tiedt TN, Albuquerque EX, Hudson CS, Rash JE. Neostigmine-induced alterations at the mammalian neuromuscular junction. I. Muscle contraction and electrophysiology. *J Pharmacol Exp Ther* 1978 May; 205 (2):326-39.

[2] Hoch W, McConville J, Helms S, Newsom-Davis J, Melms A, Vincent A. Auto-antibodies to the receptor tyrosine kinase MuSK in patients with myasthenia gravis without acetylcholine receptor antibodies. *Nat Med* 2001 Mar; 7 (3):365-8

[3] Witzemann V. Development of the neuromuscular junction. *Cell Tissue Res* 2006 Nov; 326 (2):263-71

[4] DeChiara TM, Bowen DC, Valenzuela DM, Simmons MV, Poueymirou WT, Thomas S, Kinets E, Compton DL, Rojas E, Park JS, Smith C, DiStefano PS, Glass DJ, Burden SJ, Yancopoulos GD. The receptor tyrosin kinase MuSK is required for neuromuscolar junction formation in vivo. *Cell* 1996; 85: 501–12.

[5] Hoch W, McConville J, Helms J, Newsom-Davis J, Melms A, Vincent A. Auto-antibodies to the receptor tyrosinkinase MuSK in patients with myasthenia gravis without acetylcholine receptor antibodies. *Nat Med* 2001; 7: 365–8.

[6] Selcen D, Fukuda T, Shen XM, Engel AG. Are MuSK antibodies the primary cause of myasthenic symptoms? *Neurology* 2004; 62: 1945–50

[7] Farrugia ME, Bonifati DM, Clover L, Cossins J, Beeson D, Vincent A. Effect of sera from AChR-antibody negative myasthenia gravis patients on AChR and MuSK in cell cultures. *J Neuroimmunol* 2007; 185: 136–44

[8] Le Panse R, Cizeron-Clairac G, Cuvelier M, Truffault F, Bismuth J, Nancy P, De Rosbo NK, Berrih-Aknin S. Regulatory and pathogenic mechanisms in human autoimmune myasthenia gravis. *Ann N Y Acad Sci* 2008; 1132:135-42
[9] Phillips LH, 2nd, Torner JC. Epidemiologic evidence for a changing natural history of myasthenia gravis. *Neurology* 1996 Nov; 47 (5):1233-8
[10] Flachenecker P. Epidemiology of neuroimmunological diseases. *J Neurol* 2006 Sep; 253 Suppl 5:V2-8
[11] Phillips LH, 2nd. The epidemiology of myasthenia gravis. *Ann N Y Acad Sci* 2003 Sep; 998:407-12
[12] Thanvi BR, Lo TC. Update on myasthenia gravis. *Postgrad Med J* 2004 Dec; 80 (950):690-700
[13] Myasthenia Gravis Foundation of America. Myasthenia gravis: a manual for the health care provider. 2008 [cited; Available from: http://www. myasthenia.org/docs/ MGFA_Professional Manual.pdf
[14] Scherer K, Bedlack RS, Simel DL. Does this patient have myasthenia gravis? *JAMA* 2005 Apr 20; 293 (15):1906-14
[15] Lavrnic D, Losen M, Vujic A, De Baets M, Haidukowic LJ, Stojanovic V, Trikic R, Djukic P, Apostolski S. The features of myasthenia gravis with autoantibodies to MuSK. *J Neurol Neurosurg Psychiatry* 2005; 76: 1099–102
[16] Scuderi F, Marino M, Colonna L, Mannella F, Evoli A, Provenzano C, Bartoccioni E. Anti-p110 autoantibodies identify a subtype of "seronegative" myasthenia gravis with prominent oculobulbar involvement. *Lab Invest* 2002 Sep;82(9):1139-46
[17] Evoli A, Tonali PA, Padua L, Monaco ML, Scuderi F, Batocchi AP, Marino M, Bartoccioni E. Clinical correlates with anti-MuSK antibodies in generalized seronegative myasthenia gravis. *Brain* 2003; 126: 2304–11
[18] Caress JB, Hunt CH, Batish SD. Anti-MuSK myasthenia gravis presenting with purely ocular findings. *Arch Neurol* 2005; 62: 1002–3
[19] Deymeer F, Gungor-Tuncer O, Yilmaz V, Parman Y, Serdaroglu P, Ozdemir C, Vincent A, Saruhan-Direskeneli G. Clinical comparison of anti-MuSK vs anti-AChR-positive and seronegative myasthenia gravis. *Neurology* 2007; 68: 609–11
[20] Romi F, Aarli JA, Gilhus NE. Seronegative myasthenia gravis: disease severity and prognosis. *Eur J Neurol* 2005; 12: 413–18
[21] Keesey J.C. Clinical evaluation and management of myasthenia gravis. *Muscle Nerve* 2004; 29: 484–505
[22] Evoli A, Bianchi M.R, Riso R, Minicuci G. M, Patocchi A.P, Servirei S, Scuderi F, Bartoccioni E. Response to Therapy in MuSK MG. *Ann NY Acad Sci* 2008;1132:76-83.
[23] Castleman B. The pathology of the thymus in myasthenia gravis. *Ann NY Acad Sci* 1966; 135:496-503.
[24] Marx A, Willish A, Schultz A, Gattenlöhner S, Nenninger R, Müller- Hermelink HK. Pathogenesis of myasthenia gravis. *Virchows Arch* 1997; 430: 355-364.
[25] Lauriola L, Ranelletti F, Maggiano N, Guerriero M, Punzi C, Marsili F, Bartoccioni E, Evoli A. Thymus changes in anti-MuSK-positive and -negative myasthenia gravis. *Neurology* 2005;64: 536–538.
[26] Dubowitz V, A Sewry C. Myasthenic syndromes. In: *Muscle biopsy. A practical approach.* 3rd ed. Saunders Elsevier, London. 2007: 512-515.

[27] Martignago S, Fanin M, Albertini E, Pegoraro E, Angelini C. Muscle histopathology in myasthenia gravis with antibodies against MuSK and AChR. *Neuropathol Appl Neurobiol* 2009; 35:103–110

[28] Cenacchi G, Papa V, Fanin M, Pegoraro E, Angelini C. Comparison of muscle ultrastructure in myasthenia gravis with anti-MuSK and anti-AChR antibodies. *J Neurol* 2010 Nov 19; 258:746–752.

[29] Appel SH, Anwyl R, McAdams MW, Elias S. Accelerated degradation of acetylcholine receptor from cultured rat myotubes with myasthenia gravis sera and globulins. *Proc Natl Acad Sci USA* 1977; 74: 2124–30

[30] Rostedt Punga A, Ahlqvist K, Bartoccioni E, Scuderi F, Marino M, Suomalainen A, Kalimo H, Staelberg EV. Neurophysiological and mitochondrial abnormalities in MuSK antibody seropositive myasthenia gravis compared to other immunological subtypes. *Clin Neurophysiol* 2006; 117: 1434–43.

[31] Angelini C. Diagnosis and management of autoimmune myasthenia gravis. *Clin Drug Investig.* 2011;31(1):1-14. doi: 10.2165/11584740-000000000-00000. Review

2

# Ocular Manifestations of Myasthenia Gravis

Joseph A. Pruitt and Pauline Ilsen
*Southern College of Optometry, Memphis, TN & Southern California College of Optometry, Fullerton, California*
*USA*

## 1. Introduction

Myasthenia Gravis (MG) is presently an incurable antibody-mediated autoimmune disorder characterized by generalized voluntary skeletal muscle weakness. Literally translated from its Latin and Greek etymological roots, myasthenia gravis means, "grave muscle weakness."

The cause of the weakness is due to a defect at the level of the neuromuscular junction in which autoimmune antibodies block the receptors responsible for initiating muscular contraction. The neurotransmitter that is subject to this competitive inhibition is acetylcholine (ACh). The muscles commonly affected include those of the neck, limbs and chest cavity with regards to breathing. The muscles of the eye, including those responsible for eye movements, as well as those involved with swallowing, chewing, and speaking, are most notably affected. Muscle weaknesses involving the eye produce symptoms of blurred vision, variable diplopia, and ptosis. Colavito et al. noted that nonstriated ocular muscles can also be involved in MG. They cautioned that when patients with myasthenia present with complaints of asthenopia and blur, resulting from accommodative dysfunction and vergence insufficiency, the underlying systemic disease process may be missed. Ptosis is defined as an abnormal eyelid "drooping" beyond the normal 1-2 mm of the upper limbus of the cornea.

Since the process in which the muscular weakness manifests is a result of competitive inhibition, the weakness observed is transient and improves with periods of rest. Likewise, muscular weakness increases during periods of increased or prolonged physical activity.

Even though MG is an antibody-mediated autoimmune disease, a reported 15% of patients with systemic or generalized MG have no detectable antibodies to acetylcholine receptors (i.e., they have "seronegative" MG). Seronegative MG is common in children; 40% of cases present before the age of 10 years.

It is estimated that 85-90% of all reported MG cases, whether seropositive or seronegative, present with ocular symptoms. Additionally, it has been reported that 20-50% of all cases of MG are purely ocular. Ocular myasthenia is considered a distinct diagnosis from generalized MG. Although there is evidence of ocular MG progressing to generalized MG, it has been reported that those with purely ocular symptoms for a period of 1-3 years have a greatly reduced chance of progressing on to generalized MG. Furthermore, a reported estimate of 55% of all cases of ocular MG are seropositive.

Two reasons have been suggested to explain the high proportion of MG cases that present with ophthalmic manifestations. The first is the susceptibility of ocular muscles to the disease process. The second reason is that ocular involvement in MG is relatively easy to recognize compared to that of other muscle groups. The exact reasoning why is unknown, but the following four reasons are hypothesized to contribute in part or in whole: First, even the slightest extraocular muscle (EOM) weakness will sufficiently misalign the visual axis to produce symptoms of diplopia. This is in contrast to an affected muscle in a limb, where an individual would not notice minute reductions in muscle-generated forces most likely.[7] Moreover, the ocular motor system relies primarily on visual feedback, not so much on proprioceptive mechanisms, thereby making its ability to adapt swiftly to asymmetric or variable weakness more limited compared to an extremity muscle. Second, the high firing frequencies of ocular motor neurons might contribute to neuromuscular transmission fatigue. No other motor neuron in the body exhibits the rate of firing frequency of the ocular motor neurons. It is estimated ocular motor neurons fire at a frequency exceeding up to 600 Hz during saccades. Motor neurons found elsewhere in the body rarely exceed a firing frequency of 100 Hz. Therefore, any disruption in the ability of these ocular neurons to maintain a high firing rate would cause a decrease in effectiveness and appropriate output. Myasthenia gravis produces this kind of disruption. Third, several anatomic and physiologic properties of EOM fibers make them more susceptible to neuromuscular transmission blockade. EOM nerve fibers possess anatomical characteristics that possibly make them more susceptible to neuromuscular transmission block. The fibers of the EOMs have less prominent synaptic folds, and the conclusion is drawn that there are fewer ACh receptors and sodium channels on the postsynaptic membrane. Much has been previously documented in that the mean quantal content (in other words, the average number of vesicles released during a synaptic event) of ocular motor neurons is lower than motor neurons innervating other muscles. Fourth is the preferential immunologic targeting of EOM synapses. This theory remains purely speculative, but it has been observed that the sera from some MG patients bind only to multi-innervated fibers' synapses, and the use of EOM as a source of ACh receptors for ACh antibody assays leads to higher rates of autoantibody detection, which suggests that EOMs have unique antigenic targets.

Treatment for systemic or generalized MG includes a wide variety of options, but remains primarily systemic medication. First line therapy typically consists of an acetylcholinesterase inhibitor like pyridostigmine bromide (Mestinon). Although it must be noted that pyridostigmine bromide has rather variable results in pure OMG with an approximate effectiveness ratio of 1 to 2. Another option is immunosuppressant therapy such as prednisolone, cyclosporine, azathioprine, methotrexate and mycophenolate mofetil (Cellcept). Yet again, it must be noted with regards to pure OMG, it is suggested there is not sufficient evidence to warrant the routine use of immunosuppressant therapy (i.e. corticosteroids). More drastic measures attempted in the past include systemic oral medications, plasmapheresis (a.k.a. plasma exchange) and IVIG injections. Plasmapheresis is the removal of antibodies from the blood. An IVIG injection is a sterile solution of plasma proteins containing IgG antibodies from pooled human plasma. Although the mechanism of action is unknown, it is thought to down-regulate the production of antibodies. The preparation contains no less than 90% immunoglobulin consisting of all the IgG substances and trace amount of IgA and IgM. However, this treatment is usually reserved for patients demonstrating dysphagia with an associated high risk of aspiration and those who are unable to ambulate without assistance. Although slower-acting than plama exchange, the response is similar and offers advantages when therapeutic plasmaphesis is not available or when vascular access is problematic. Significant improvement is seen in patients whose therapy consist of an initial dose of 400 mg/kg/d for 5 days and followed by maintenance with 400 mg/kg once monthly. Furthermore, it has been noted that with regards to a similarly treated disease, Guillian-Epstein Barr Syndrome, IVIG treatment in many ways is considered to be the more effective successor to plasmapheresis.

Thymectomy, the surgical removal of the thymus gland, is also an effective and accepted treatment for generalized MG; however, while effective, it is controversial as a treatment measure in pure OMG. Recent theories suggest thymectomies could be performed on early presentations of OMG to prevent and/or slow the disease progression and immunosuppressive therapy only if proven necessary. Thymectomies are often performed on young individuals in the early stages of MG regardless of the presence of a tumor.[8] As related to generalized MG and post-surgical improvement, it has been shown both the grade of follicular hyperplasia and density of T-cell subsets in the middle part of the thymus (space between the superior and inferior horns) had a significant correlation with the level of improvement of MG after thymectomy.

Additionally, if there is found to be thyroid involvement, a throidectomy is a viable treatment option.

Treatment for ocular MG specifically may include all the aforementioned options because a report 50-60% of individuals who present with purely ocular MG will eventually progress and develop generalize MG. Nevertheless, ocular MG treatments consist of both surgical and non-surgical treatments. Surgical options for myogenic ptosis are ptosis repair surgery, blepharoplasty, and frontalis suspension for which a Tutoplast sling can be utilized, external levator advancement, and tarsomyectomy. A non-surgical option is Botulinum Toxin Type A (Botox) injection to temporarily treat myogenic ptosis.

The first line of treatment should be a refraction in order to achieve the patient's best corrected visual acuity (BCVA). Assessment of accmodation and vergence testing should also be considered. As for diplopia, standard treatments such as occlusion and prisms are commonly employed. However, with prisms, the practitioner must keep in mind the variability of the disease's manifestations, thereby making it possible for the angle of deviation to fluctuate.

## 2. References

Rowland R, Sparr S. Head-drop and shortness of breath as a presentation of myasthenia gravis. J Am Geriatr Soc 2007;55(4):S116

Palace J, Vincnet A, Beeson D. Myasthenia gravis: diagnostic and management dilemmas. Current Opinion in Neurology 2001;14:583-589

Homel P, Kupersmith M. Development of Generalized Myasthenia Gravis in Patinets With Ocular Myasthenia Gravis. Arch Neurol 2003; 60(10):1491-1492

Hilton-Jones D, Palace J. The management of myasthenia gravis. Practical Neurology 2005;5:18-27

http://www.ninds.nih.gov/disorders/myasthenia_gravis/myasthenia_gravis.htm
Golnik K. How to Diagnose and Treat Myasthenia Gravis. Review of Ophthalmology. 2002;9(10):219.
Ubogu E, Kaminski H. The Preferential Involvement of Extraocular Muscle by Myasthenia Gravis. Neuro-ophthalmology, 2001;25(4):219-228
Colavito J, Cooper J, Ciuffreda K. Non-ptotic ocular myasthenia gravis: a common presentation of an uncommon disease. Optometry. 76(7): 363-375.
Cameron R, Loehrer P, Thomas C. Thymic Neoplasms; Neoplasms of the Mediastinum. Principles & Practice of Oncology 7th Edition. Chapter 28. Lippincott Williams & Wilkins. 2005.
Donati F, Bevan D. Neuromuscular Blocking Agents. Clinical Anesthesia 5th Edition. Chapter 16. Lippincott Williams & Wilkins. 2006.
Toyka K. Ptosis in myasthenia gravis: Extended fatigue and recovery bedside test. Neurology 2006;67(8):1524
Reddy A, Backhouse O. "Ice-on-eyes", a simple test for myasthenia gravis presenting with ocular symptoms. Practical Neurology 2007;7(2):109-111
Benatar M, Kaminski H. Evidence report: The medical treatment of ocular myasthenia (an evidence-based review): Report of the Quality Standards Subcommittee of the American Academy of Neurology. Neurology 2007;68(24):2144-2149
Rudnicki S. Lamber-Eaton Myasthenic Syndrome with Pure Ocular Weakness. Neurology 2007;68(21):1863-1864
Lapid O. Eyelid Crutches for Ptosis: A Forgotten Solution. Plastic and Reconstructive Surgery. October 2000. 106(5): 1213-1214.
Scherer K, Bedlack R, Simel D. Does This Patient Have Myasthenia Gravis?. JAMA 2005;293(15):1906-1914
Morris O, O'day J. Fatiguable Ptosis and Pseudoretraction Caused by Myasthenia Gravis. Clinical and Experimental Ophthalmology. 2004; 32:303-304
Shaw J. When Muscles Falter: Update on Myasthenia Gravis. Clinical Update: Neuro-opthalmology; http://www.aao.org/publications/eyenet/200607/neuro.cfm. 2006
Golnik K, Pena R, Lee A, Eggenberger R. An Ice Test for the Diagnosis of Myasthenia Gravis. Ophthalmology. 1999; 106(7): 1282-1286
Kennard C. Examine eye movements. Practical Neurology 2007;7:326-330 Tomelleri G, Vattemi G, Filosto M, Tonin P. Eyelid ptosis from sympathetic nerve dysfunction mistaken as myopathy: a simple test to identify this condition. J Neurol Neurosurg Psychiatry 2007;78(6):632-634
Chan J, Orrison W. Ocular Myasthenia: A Rare Presentation with MuSK
Antibody and Bilateral Extraocular Muscle Atrophy. Br. J. Ophthalmol. 2007;91:842-843
Kubis K, Danesh-Meyer H, Savino P, Sergott R. The Ice Test versus the Rest Test in Myasthenia Gravis. Ophthalmology. 2000;107(11): 1995-1998
Gilbert M, De Sousa E, Savino P, Peter J. Ocular Myasthenia Gravis Treatment: The Case Against Prednisone Therapy and Thymectomy. Archives of Neurology. December 2007. 64(12): 1790-1792.
Chavis P, Stickler D, Walker A. Immunosuppressive or Surgical Treatment for Ocular Myasthenia Gravis. Archives of Neurology. December 2007. 64(12): 1792-1794.

Kupersmith M, Latkany R, Homel P. Development of Generalized Disease at 2 Years in Patients With Ocular Myasthenia Gravis. Archives of Neurology. February 2003. 60(2): 243-248.

Kaminski H, Daroff R. Treatment of Ocular Myasthenia: Steroids Only When Compelled. Archives of Neurology. May 2000. 57(5): 752-753

Bennett D, Mills K, Riordan-Eva P, Barnes P, Rose M. Anti-MuSK antibodies in a case of ocular myasthenia gravis. Journal of Neurology, Neurosurgery, & Psychiatry. April 2006. 77(4): 564-565.

Caress J, Hunt C, Batish S. Anti-MuSK Myasthenia Gravis Presenting With Purely Ocular Findings. Archives of Neurology. June 2005. 62(6): 1002-1003.

Elrod RD, Weinberg DA. Ocular myasthenia gravis. *Ophthalmol Clin North Am* 2004 Sep;17(3):275-309.

Sommer N, Sigg B, Melms A, Weller M, Schepelmann K, Herzau V, Dichgans J. Ocular myasthenia gravis: response to long term immunosuppressive treatment. J Neurol Neurosurg Psychiatry 1997;62(2):156-162

Howard J. Intravenous Immunoglobulin for the Treatment of Acquired Myasthenia Gravis. Neurology. December 1998. 51(6) Supplement 5: S30-S36.

http://www.umd.nycpic.com/cgi-bin/bookmgr/bookmgr.exe/BOOKS/D971-2A/FRONT

Hilkevich O, Drory V, Chapman J, Korczyn A. The Use of Intravenous Immunoglobulin as Maintenance Therapy in Myasthenia Gravis. Clinical Neuropharmacology. May/June 2001. 24(3): 173-176.

Meche F, Schmitz P. A Randomized Trial Comparing Intravenous Immune Globulin and Plasma Exchange in Guillian-Barre Syndrome. Dutch Guillian-Barre Study Group. The New England Journal of Medicine. 1992(17); 326:1123-1129.

Roberts P, Venuta F, Rendina E, De Giacomo T, Coloni G, Follette D, Richman D, Benfield J. Thymectomy in the treatment of ocular myasthenia gravis. The Journal of Thoracic and Cardiovascular Surgery. September 2001. 122(3): 562-568.

Lauriola L, Ranelletti F, Maggiano N, Guerriero M, Punzi C, Marsili F, Bartoccioni E, Evoli A. Thymus changes in anti-MuSK-positive and –negative myasthenia gravis. Neurology. 8 February 2005. 64(3): 536-538.

Agius M. Treatment of Ocular Myasthenia With Corticosteroids: Yes. Archives of Neurology. May 2000. 57(4): 750-751.

Mori T, Nomori H, Ikeda K, Kobayashi H, Iwatani K, Kobayashi T. The distribution of parenchyma, follicles, and lymphocyte subsets in thymus of patients with myasthenia gravis, with special reference to remission after thymectomy. The Journal of Thoracic and Cardiovascular Surgery. February 2007. 133(2): 364-368.

Periman L, Sires B. Floppy Eyelid Syndrome: A Modified Surgical Technique. Ophthalmic Plastic and Reconstructive Surgery 2002;18(5):370-372Sakol P, Mannor G, Massaro B. Congenital and acquired blepharoptosis. Current Opinion in Ophthalmology 1999;10:335-339Lauriola L, Ranelletti F, Maggiano N, Guerriero M, Punzi C, Marsili F, Bartoccioni E, Evoli A. Thymus changes in anti-MuSK-positive and –negative myasthenia gravis. Neurology. 8 February 2005. 64(3): 536-538.

Shields M, Putterman A. Blepharoptosis correction. Current Opinion in Otolaryngology & Head and Neck Surgery 2003;11(4):261-266

Sakol P, Mannor G, Massaro B. Congenital and acquired blepharoptosis. Current Opinion in Ophthalmology 1999;10:335-339

Eliasoph I. RE: "Surgical Correction of Blepharoptosis in Patients with Myasthenia Gravis". Opththal Plast Reconstr Surg 2002;18(4): 312-313

McCord C, Seify H, Codner M. Transblepharoplasty Ptosis Repair: Three-Step Technique. Plastic and Reconstructive Surgery 2007;120(4):1037-1044

Seider N, Beiran I, Kaltreider S. One medial triangular Tutoplast sling as a frontalis suspension for adult myogenic blepharoptosis. Acta Ophthalmologica Scandinavica 2006;84:121-123

Wong, V, Beckingsale P, Olley C, Sullivan T. Management of Myogenic Ptosis. Ophthalmology. 2002;109(5): 1023-1031

Bernardini F, Concillis C, Devoto M. Frontalis Suspension Sling using a Silicone Rod in Patients affected by Myogenic Blepharoptosis. Orbit. 2002; 21(3): 195-198

Gausas R, Goldstein S. Ptosis in the Elderly Patient. Int Ophthalmol Clin 2002;42(2):61-74

Bradley E, Bartley G, Chapman K, Waller R. Surgical Correction of Blepharoptosis in Patients With Myasthenia Gravis. Ophthalmic Plastic and Reconstructive Surgery. March 2001. 17(2): 103-110.

Morris O, O'Day J. Strabismus Surgery in the Management of Diplopia caused by Myasthenia Gravis. Br. J. Ophthalmol. 2004; 88: 832-850

Takagi S, Hosokawa K, Yano K, Kunihiro N, Tateki K. Crutches Glasses For Blepharoptosis. Plastic and Reconstructive Surgery. June 2002. 109(7): 2605

Frueh BR. The mechanistic classification of ptosis. *Ophthalmol* 1980; 87(10):1019-21.

# Part 2

## Treatments

# 3

# Myasthenia Gravis – Current Treatment Standards and Emerging Drugs

Kamil Musilek[1,2,3*], Marketa Komloova[4], Ondrej Holas[4], Anna Horova[1], Jana Zdarova-Karasova[3,5] and Kamil Kuca[3,6]
[1]*University of Defence, Faculty of Military Health Sciences, Department of Toxicology, Hradec Kralove*
[2]*University of Hradec Kralove, Faculty of Science Department of Chemistry, Hradec Kralove*
[3]*Centre for Biomedical Research, University Hospital, Hradec Kralove*
[4]*Charles University in Prague, Faculty of Pharmacy in Hradec Kralove, Department of Pharmaceutical Chemistry and Drug Control, Hradec Kralove*
[5]*University of Defence, Faculty of Military Health Sciences, Department of Public Health, Hradec Kralove*
[6]*University of Defence, Faculty of Military Health Sciences, Center of Advanced Studies, Hradec Kralove*
*Czech Republic*

## 1. Introduction

Myasthenia gravis is very rare disorder resulting from the autoimmune destruction of postsynaptic membrane in neuromuscular junction. In the most cases, antibodies bind to nicotinic acetylcholine receptors (nAChR), although other structures (e.g. muscle specific tyrosin kinase; MuSK) can be targeted as well. Binding antibody initiates immunological attack leading to reduced density of nAChR, simplification of the membrane and consequently to impaired neuromuscular transmission (Santa 1972). Clinical manifestation of the disease is described as fatiguable weakness of the striated muscles, which is painless and usually worsen after exercise. Initial symptom is asymmetrical ptosis of the upper eyelids frequently accompanied by the diplopia or blurred vision. An extension to another facial muscle groups can lead to expressionless appearance and difficulties with swallowing, chewing and speaking. The disease has a progressive character and it may become generalized after some time. The severe cases of MG require close monitoring of patient vital functions, because the risk of dyspnoea arises with the weakness of the intercostal muscles and diaphragm (Thanvi 2004).

Myasthenia gravis, formerly a lethal disease, may be now effectively treated, returning patient back to normal life. Nowadays, the treatment can be individualized to every patient according to the age and co-morbidities thanks to the wide variety of drugs available for different form and severity of the disease. Different approaches in the treatment strategy and possibility of combining them also allow minimization of the adverse effects.

## 2. Acetylcholinesterase inhibitors

Acetylcholinesterase inhibitors (AChEIs) were first introduced to the clinical practice by Mary B. Walker in 1930's. She studied the similarities in the symptoms of curare poisoning and Myasthenia gravis during administration of physostigmine (curare antidote). She observed a temporary improvement in the muscle weakness of MG patient (Walker 1934).

AChEIs still remain the first-line treatment in the initial stages or in the mild forms of the disease. They are also administered to the patients, who experience residual weakness, while using immunotherapy or those, who cannot receive immunosuppressive treatment (Juel 2007). AChEI slow down the degradation of acetylcholine (ACh) by acetylcholinesterase (AChE; Fig. 1). They increase ACh levels in the synaptic cleft and thus enhance impaired cholinergic transmission presuming that there is sufficient amount of the nicotinic acetylcholine receptors (AChR) left (Richman 2003). However, they provide only symptomatic treatment and do not modify the underlying progress of the disease.

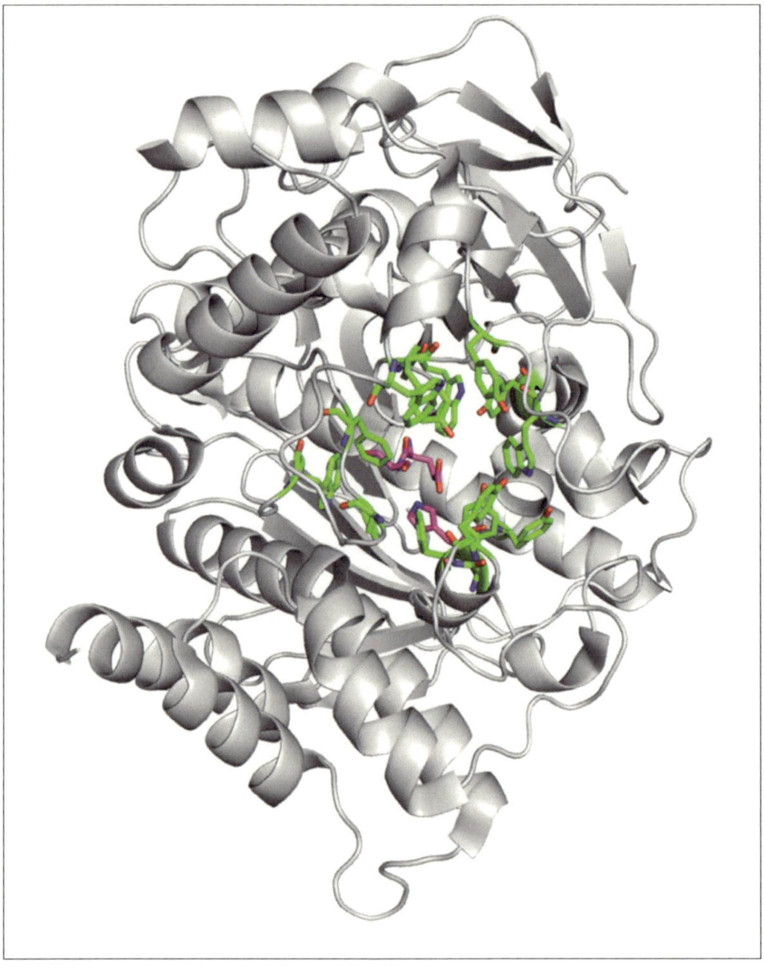

Fig. 1. Human recombinant acetylcholinesterase (1b41.pdb) with important aromatic residues (in green) and catalytic triade (in magenta).

Peripheral AChEI currently used in the therapy of MG are charged molecules usually containing one or two quaternary nitrogen in their structure. Most of them are derived from carbamic acids (pyridostigmine bromide, neostigmine bromide, distigmine dibromide). The non-carbamate bisquaternary drug ambenonium dichloride is structurally distinct representative of AChEI, and it has one of the highest affinities to AChE (Hodge 1992).

Effective dosing must be individualized to each patient according to his age, gender and eventual co-morbidities. Gastrointestinal side effects are related to the increased muscarinic activity produced by mentioned drugs and include nausea, vomiting, abdominal cramping and diarrhea. They can be treated with antimuscarinics (loperamide hydrochloride, diphenoxylate hydrochloride, propantheline bromide) without the loss of nicotinic effect (Hill 2003, Thanvi 2004). High doses of AChEI can lead to a cholinergic crisis characterized by even greater muscular weakness accompanied by increased bronchial secretion, diarrhea, abdominal pain, hypersalivation and bradycardia (Juel 2007; Thanvi 2004; Garcia-Carrasco 2007).

## 2.1 Pyridostigmine

Pyridostigmine (Mestinon®, Regonol®, Fig. 2; Urban 1951) Pyridostigmine bromide is the most globally used AChEI in the MG treatment. It is generally better tolerated than neostigmine bromide and has fewer gastrointestinal side effects (Juel 2005). The dosing often starts at 30 mg of pyridostigmine three times a day and can be increased up to 90 mg three or four times a day. The improvement in muscle strength usually develops 30 minutes after ingestion and lasts for four hours (Juel 2007).

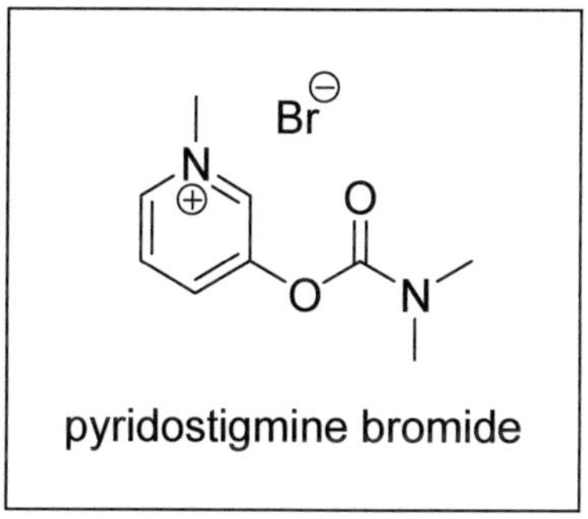


Fig. 2. Pyridostigmine bromide.

## 2.2 Neostigmine

Neostigmine (Prostigmine®, Vagostigmine®, Fig. 3; Aeschlimann 1933) has a rapid onset but its effect lasts only 2-3 hours. It is prescribed for patients with ocular MG. It is possible to administer neostigmine intravenously or subcutaneously, if the patient is experiencing difficulties with swallowing. More recently, a nasal application was successfully tested (Sghirlanzoni 1992).

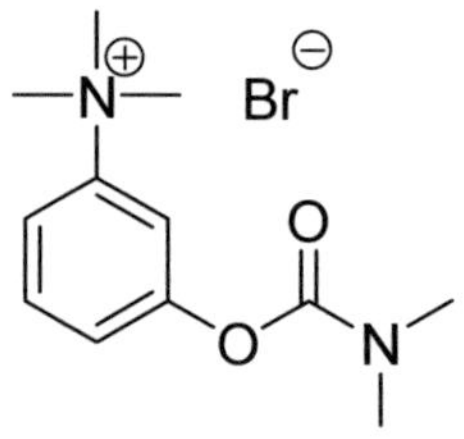

neostigmine bromide

Fig. 3. Neostigmine bromide

### 2.3 Distigmine

Distigmine (Ubretid®, Fig. 4; Schmid 1957) is AChEI with prolonged effect (12-16 hours). It is used by patients without fluctuating physical exercise usually twice a day in the dose of 5 mg. Its prolonged effect is used for the patients experiencing the morning weakness, when it is administered in the evening the day before (Haward 1990).

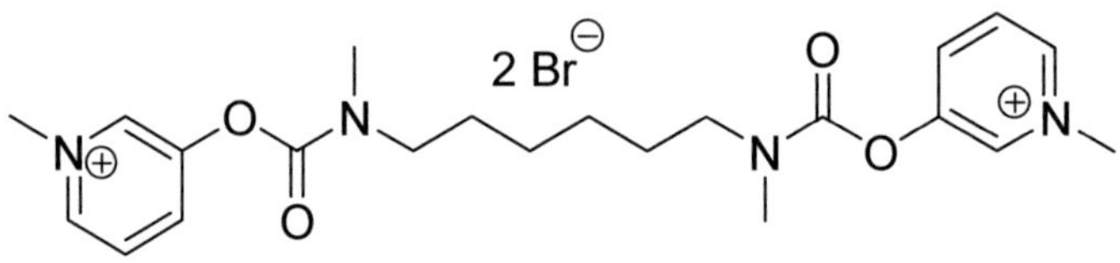

distigmine dibromide

Fig. 4. Distigmine dibromide

### 2.4 Ambenonium

Ambenonium dichloride (Mytelase®, Fig. 5; Kirchner 1958) is AChEI with slower onset and prolonged pharmacological effect. It can improve clinical state of the patient, who has received other AChEI for a long time. The dosing is very individual and is usually 3-4 times a day up to 10 mg. Its side effects manifest very inconspicuously and cholinergic crises can be very dramatic (Verma 1992).

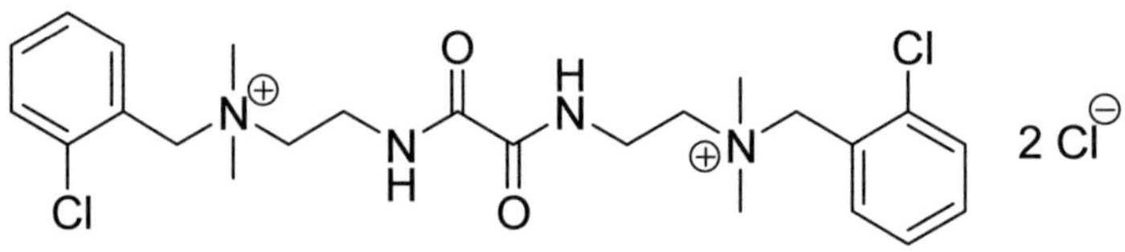

ambenonium dichloride

Fig. 5. Ambenonium dichloride.

### 2.5 Novel peripherally acting AChEIs

Despite the clinically used AChEI, there are many other peripherally acting AChEI with possible use for early MG stages (Komloova 2010). Many of such compounds were developed during the last decade. For this MG purposes, edrophonium like AChE inhibitors were prepared and they valuably showed sub-nanomolar AChE inhibition (Leonetti 2008). The bis-pyridinium heterodimers also proved high inhibitory potential (nanomolar range) and selectivity towards AChE compared to butyrylcholinesterase or choline kinase (Conejo-Garcia 2011). Similarly, the bis-pyridinium, bis-quinolonium and bis-isoquinolinium homodimers presented high AChE inhibiton (nanomolar range) and some of them improved selectivity towards AChE (Musilek 2010, Musilek 2011, Komloova 2011). Such compounds might become the aim of further interest after essential *in vitro* and *in vivo* evaluation and they might lack the side effects of currently used AChEIs.

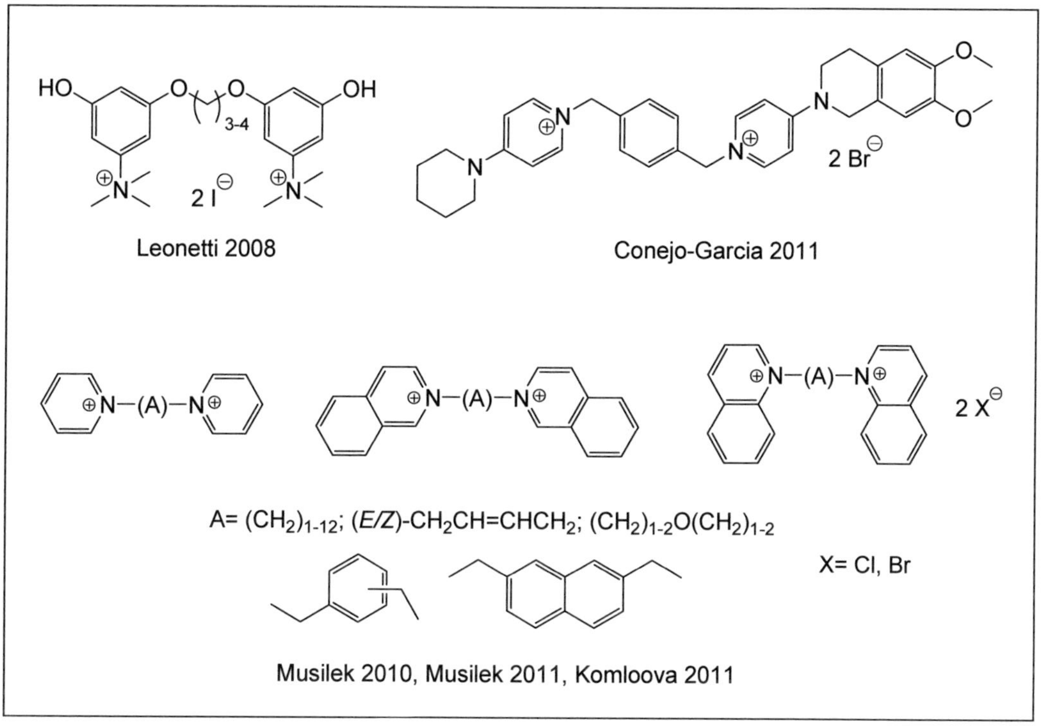


Fig. 6. Novel AChEIs tested for possible MG use.

## 3. Corticosteroids

Since a corticosteroid treatment is efficient in many autoimmune diseases, they are also used in the MG treatment, although their mechanism of action is not fully explained (Schneider-Gold 2005). Their interference with the immune system leads to anti-inflammatory, anti-allergic and anti-proliferative effect. Additionally, an increased expression and stabilization of acetylcholine receptors was observed in a long term administration of corticosteroids (Braun 1993). The corticosteroids belong to the standard treatment of MG moderate forms and MG mild forms insufficiently responding to the treatment with AChEIs.

The administration of corticosteroids is very often connected to the large amount of the adverse effects that are dose-dependent and may become very serious. For these reasons, it is important to minimize effective steroid dose individually for each patient. The side effects developed during corticosteroid treatment are metabolic disorders (hyperlipidemia, diabetes mellitus and potassium loss), hypertension, gastric ulceration, osteoporosis, cataracts, glaucoma, reduced immunity, muscle atrophy or psychic disorders (Juel 2007).

### 3.1 Prednisone

Prednisone (Decortin®, Encorton®, Fig. 6; Oliveto 1959) is the most used corticosteroid for MG treatment. There are two known approaches in its dosing strategy. The first approach starts with high daily dose of prednisone (from 1.5 -2.0 mg/kg/day or 60-80 mg/day), which is maintained for 2 -4 weeks and the dosing is modified to alternate day schedule (100-120 mg every other day) after the sufficient muscle improvement. The dose is then gradually decreased to minimize the side effects, while there is still satisfactory response in the muscle strength (Juel 2005). The reduction of the steroid dosage must be performed slowly and adequately to the responses of the patient, because the myasthenic relapse can occur and a rapid withdrawal of the steroid may result into myasthenic exacerbation and crisis (Juel 2007). Consequently, the dose reduction is performed in 4-8 week intervals from 10 mg to 30 mg/alternate day and then from 5 mg to 20 mg/alternate day (Juel 2005). Some patients do not tolerate this alternate-day schedule, because of the mood instability or difficult glycaemia control in the case of diabetic patients (Juel 2007). This alternate-day treatment may also require additional immunosuppressive treatment in the days without corticosteroids.

The second approach starts with 10-20 mg/day and increases the dose by 5-10 mg/week up to maximum dose of 50-60 mg/day until the satisfactory improvement in the muscle strength occurs. The dose is then gradually reduced to minimize the side effects (Schwendimann 2005, Seybold 1974, Sghirlanzoni 1984).

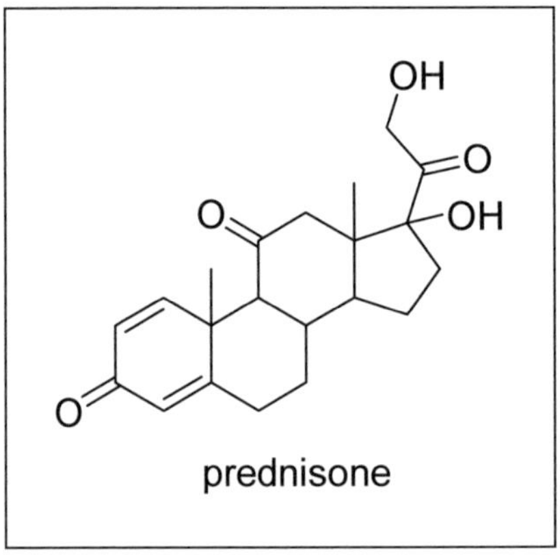


Fig. 6. Prednisone.

## 4. Immunosuppressants

Long-term corticosteroid treatment is usually connected with many serious dose-dependent side effects. Conventional immunosuppressants are used in MG to help to avoid these corticosteroid side effects. They act more selectively on specific phases of the cell cycle. Azathioprine, cyclophosphamide, cyclosporine, mycophenolate mofetil and tacrolimus are the most utilized immunosuppressants in the MG treatment. They can be combined together, or with glucocorticosteroids, allowing reduction of corticosteroid doses and thus minimizing the side effects. If used in monotherapy, it takes a certain time before the effect of these drugs is manifested. It is therefore recommended to start the immunosuppressive treatment along with corticosteroids and then gradually reduce the corticosteroid dosing.

### 4.1 Azathioprine

Azathioprine (Imuran®, Azamun®, Fig. 7) is the most often used steroid-sparing immunosuppressant (Hitchings 1962). It has few side effects and it is generally better tolerated in the long-term treatment compared to corticosteroids (Kokontis 2000). Azathioprine is an anti-metabolite. After ingestion, it is metabolized into 6-mercaptopurine, which is an inhibitor of purine synthesis and subsequently proliferation of rapid growing cells, especially lymphocytes (Juel 2007). The initial dose is 50 mg/day partially increased every week into optimal treatment dose of 2-2.5 mg/kg/day (Saperstein 2004, Schwendimann 2005). Application of azathioprine in combination with prednisone was found very advantageous thanks to slow onset of azathioprine effect. This combination also allowed the reduced dosing of both drugs (Gajdos 1983, Mantegazza 1988).

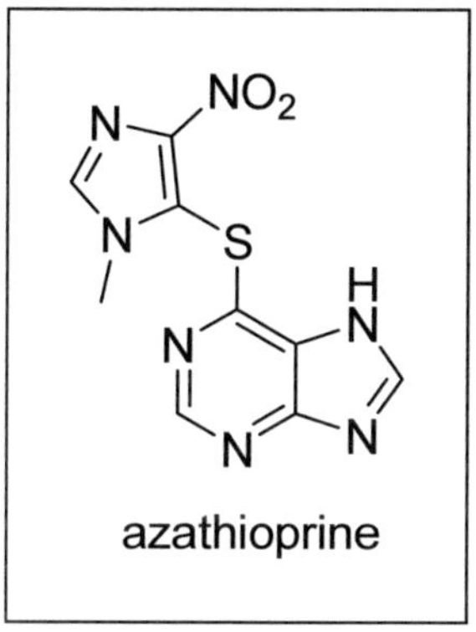


Fig. 7. Azathioprine.

Side effects of azathioprine consist in hepatotoxicity, myelo-suppression, potential carcinogenesis and teratogenesis, rarely alopecia and increased risk of lymphoma after long-term use (Herrllinger 2000). In 10-15% patients, an idiosyncratic allergy with rush, fever, nausea, vomiting and abdominal pain can occur (Hohlfeld 1988, Kissel 1986).

### 4.2 Cyclophosphamide

Cyclophosphamide (Cyclophosphamid®, Fig. 8; Arnold 1958) is a cytostatic drug with the alkylating mechanism of action used primarily in the treatment of cancer (Zhu 1987). It is metabolized by hepatic oxidases into phosphoramide mustard, active form of cyclophosphamide, responsible for its alkylating and cytotoxic properties. Cyclophosphamide is very toxic agent with terratogenic, carcinogenic and myelotoxic side effects. It may also cause hemorrhagic cystitis and sterility (Richman 2003). It is reserved for patients with severe forms of MG and in combination with corticosteroids for those, who do not respond adequately to the treatment with corticosteroids alone (De Feo 2002). Common dosing is 100-200 mg daily.

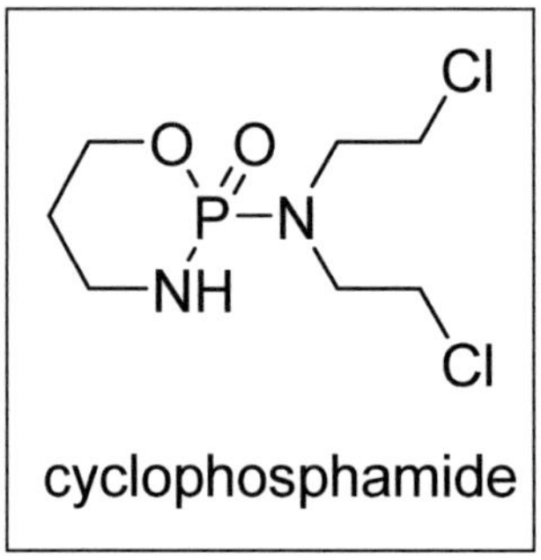


Fig. 8. Cyclophosphamide.

#### 4.3 Cyclosporine

Cyclosporine (Sandimun®, Consupren®, Fig. 9) is a cyclic polypeptide produced by *Tolypocladium terricola* (Hassan 1987). His high nefrotoxicity and numerous interactions with other drugs make it a second choice immunosuppressant, reserved for patients with generalized severe MG form refractory to conventional treatment (Kahan 1989, Nyberg-Hnasen 1988).

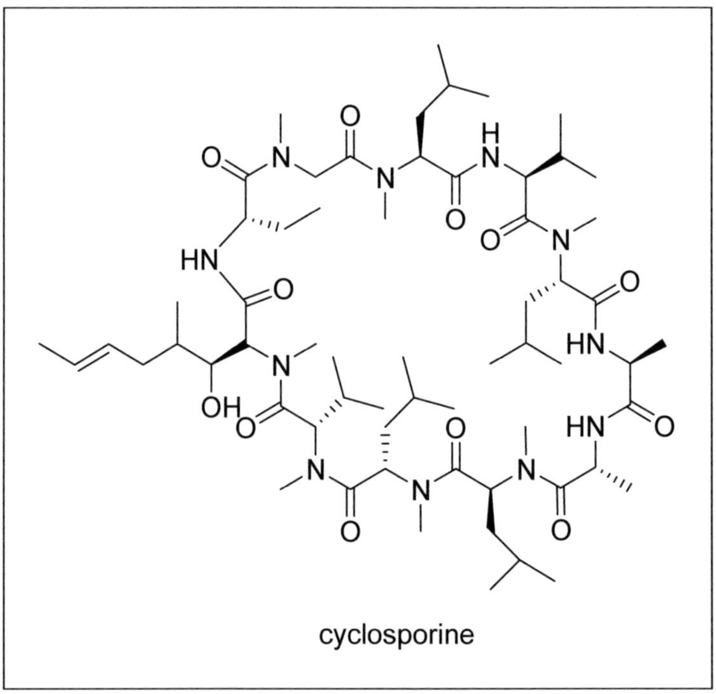


Fig. 9. Cyclosporine.

Cyclosporine affects T-lymphocytes and inhibits production of IL-2 and other cytokines (Matzuda 2000). A randomized double-blind placebo-controlled study showed significant MG improvement in muscle strength upon the usage of cyclosporine (Tindall 1993). Standard cyclosporine dosage is 2.5 mg/kg every 12 hours to achieve serum level of 100-150 µg/liter. The monitoring of cyclosporine levels in serum is required to maintain the therapeutic concentration and prevent nefrotoxicity. Apart from nefrotoxicity, cyclosporine produces other side effects such as hypertension, tremor, hirsuteness, headaches, nausea and gingival hypertrophy (Juel 2005). Recent studies also suggest that cyclosporine may induce carcinogenesis by the direct cellular mechanism including production of transformed β-growth factor (TGF-β; Hojo 1999).

### 4.4 Tacrolimus

Tacrolimus (Prograf®, Advagraf®, Fig. 10) is a relatively new found macrolide immunosuppressant isolated from *Streptomyces tsukubaensis* (Okuhara 1986, Kino 1987). Likewise cyclosporine A, tacrolimus affects T-lymphocytes through calcium-calcineurin pathway inhibiting production of inflammatory cytokines, e.g. IL-2, IL-3, IL-4, IL-5 and TNF-α (Kawaguchi 2007). Immunosuppressant abilities of Tacrolimus have already been used successfully in the prevention of rejection of transplanted organs (Vincenti 2001) and treatment of other autoimmune disorders, e.g. systemic lupus erythematosus (Duddridge 1997, Solsky 2002) and rheumatoid arthritis (Gremillion 1999).

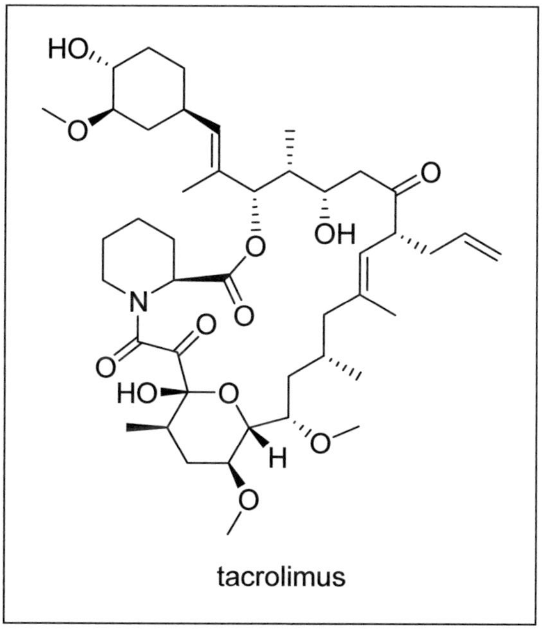


Fig. 10. Tacrolimus.

*In vitro* studies have also suggested that tacrolimus may enhance the effect of corticosteroids (Yang-Min 1993) allowing the reduction of doses in the steroid-dependent patients. Pharmacokinetic properties are highly individual for each patient and the dosage must be titrated in order to maximize the effect. It is usually administered orally in a dose of 3 mg/day and subsequently titrated to achieve blood levels of 10 ng/ml (Yang-Min 1993). Associated adverse effects are neurotoxicity, nefrotoxicity, impaired glucose metabolism (hyperglycemia through the reduction of insulin secretion; Nevins 2000), gastrointestinal discomforts and hypertension (Mayer 1997).

### 4.5 Mycophenolate mofetil

Mycophenolate mofetil (CellCept®, Fig. 11) was originally designed to prevent rejection of transplanted organs, but additionally it became very useful in the treatment of many autoimmune diseases. It is a prodrug of mycophenolic acid (Alsberg 1912), antibiotic compound produced by *Penicillium brevi-compactum, P. stoloniferum* and related spp. Its mechanism of action consist in the blockade of purine nucleotides synthesis and consequently the inhibition of lymphocyte proliferation. It also helps to increased apoptosis of lymphocytes and monocytes (Cohn 1999) and reduces the secretion of immunoglobulines and inflammatory cytokines (Durez 1999, Eugui 1991). Its benefit in the MG treatment was demonstrated in many clinical trials (Chaudhry 2001, Ciafaloni 2001, Hauser 1998, Meriggioli 2003). However, its use is reserved for the patients with severe MG refractory to combination of corticosteroid/azathioprine treatment with standard dose of 1-1.5g twice a day (Juel 2005).

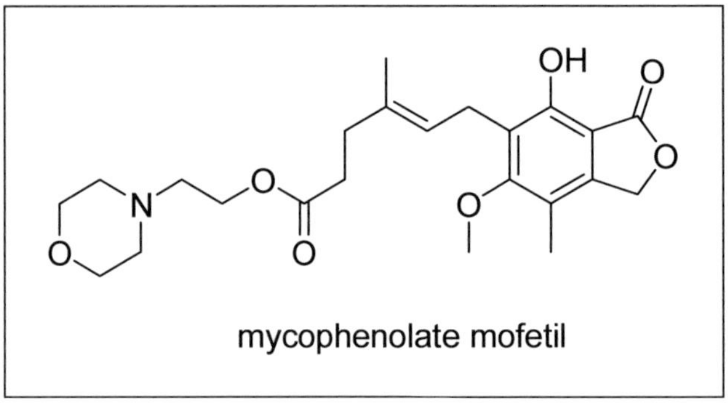


Fig. 11. Mycophenolate mofetil.

## 5. Biological treatment

The possibility of using products of immune system in the treatment of diseases was first mentioned by German scientist Paul Ehrlich in the beginning of 20th century. It took further 100 years, when an immunologic procedure could be involved in the practice. An important invention connected with progress in biological treatment was the discovery of preparation procedure for monoclonal antibodies by Caesar Milstein, Niels Kaj Jerne and George F. Köhler in 1975. Other representatives in the group of biological therapeutics apart from monoclonal antibodies are fusion proteins and the products of genome engineering designed to modify immunological response of the organism. These drugs are usually well tolerated and they offer advantageous alternative to conventional immuno-treatment (Sobotkova 2008).

### 5.1 Etanercept

Etanercept (Enbrel®, Fig. 12) is a fusion protein (Smith 1994, Jacobs 1997). These fusion or chimeric proteins are created by the connection of two genes coding originally two different proteins. Fusion protein combines properties of both original proteins. Etanercept is consisted from the human soluble receptor for tumor necrosis factor (TNF) linked to Fc portion of human immunoglobulin $G_1$. Its dimeric structure increases its affinity to TNF-α. Its mechanism of action consists in the inhibition of the biological effect of TNF. Etanercept is administered subcutaneously 1-2 a week (Rovin 2008).

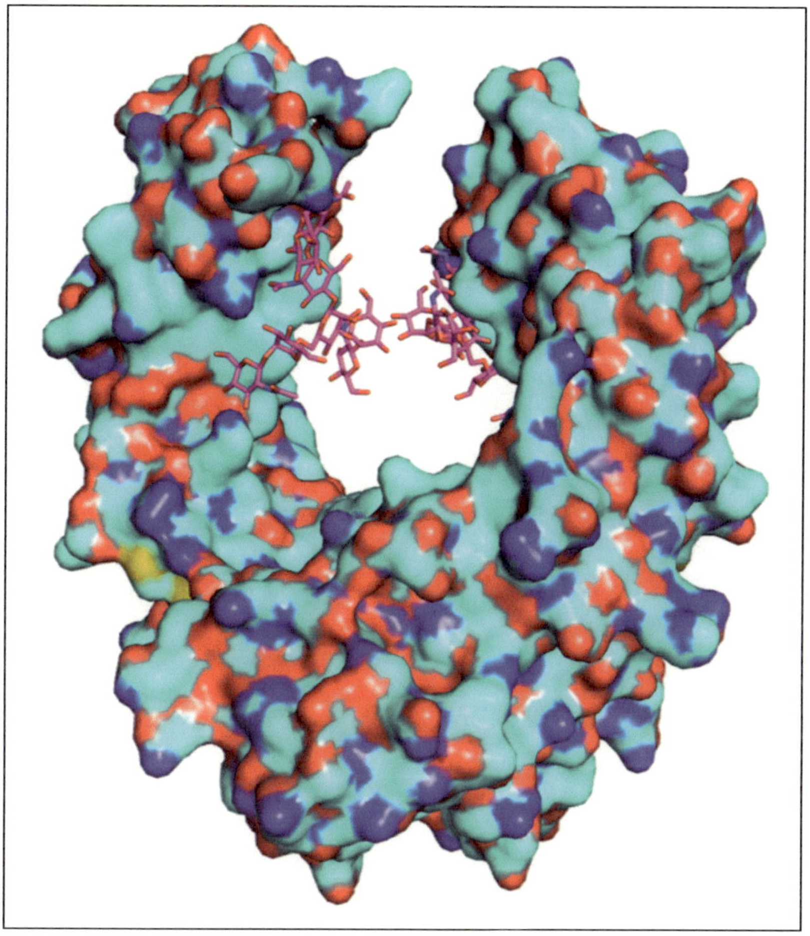

Fig. 12. Etanercept.

### 5.2 Rituximab

Rituximab (Rituxan®, MabThera®, Fig. 13) is a genetically engineered chimeric murine-human monoclonal antibody directed against the CD20 antigen found on B-lymphocyte surface (Anderson 1994, Anderson 1998). The application of rituximab leads to depletion of B-lymphocytes, while other blood elements remain intact. After its use, the levels of serum immunoglobulines were minimally decreased. This finding led to assumption that the reduction of the immunoglobulin production is not the main mechanism of action in the treatment of autoimmune diseases. The drug is usually administered in the intravenous infusion. During the infusion, the rituximab rigor, fever and hypotension can develop as a result of released cytokines. More severe, but rare side effects are hypoxia and cardiovascular collapse (Yazici 2007; Eisenberg 2005).

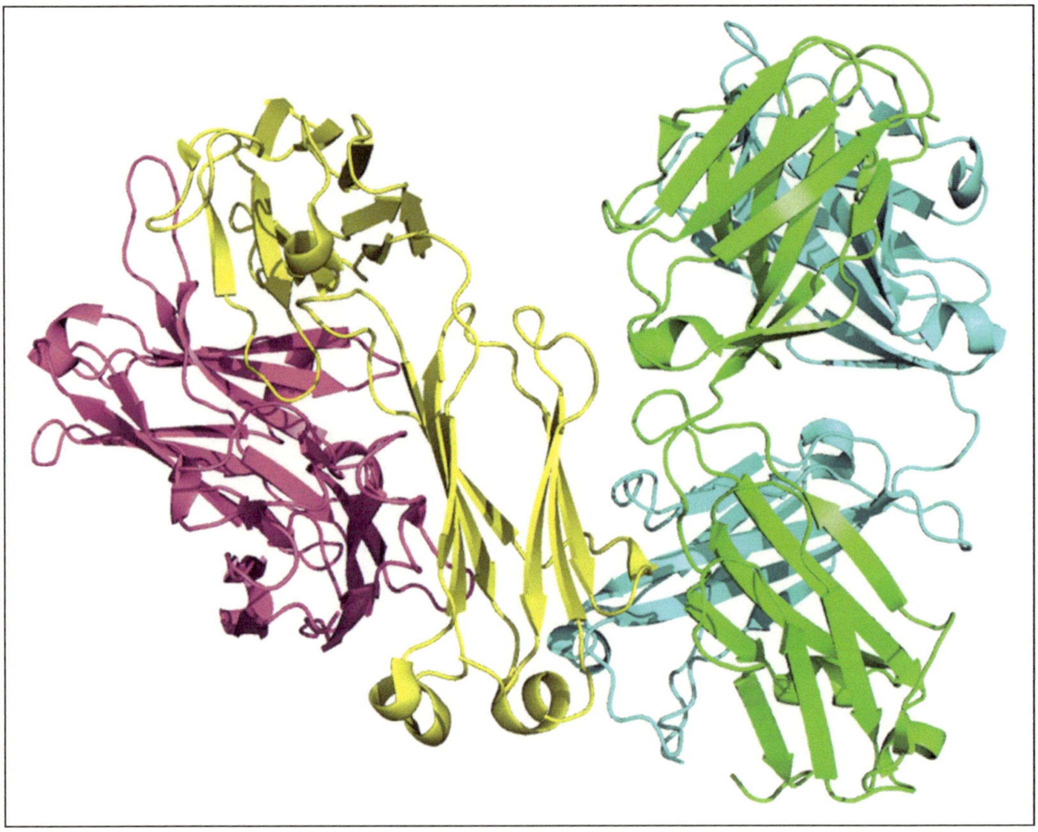

Fig. 13. Rituximab.

### 5.3 Basiliximab

Basiliximab (Simulect®, Fig. 14) is a human-murine chimeric monoclonal antibody directed against IL-2 receptor (CD25) antigen on the surface of T-lymphocytes (Amlot 1991). It is administered intravenously in a short infusion and its effect lasts for 4-6 weeks. There is the enhanced risk of anaphylactic reaction during the application of basiliximab. Other side effects are headaches, anemia, hypertension, obstipation, diarrhea, nausea and infections (Pascual 2001; Kakoulidou 2008).

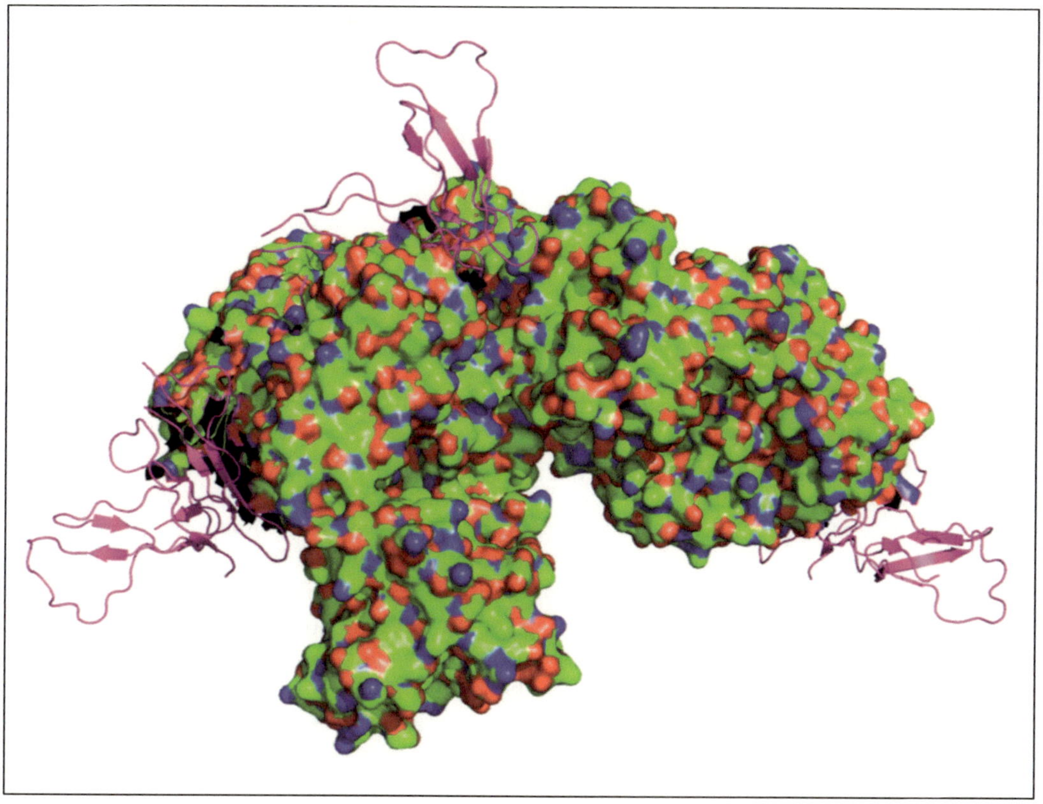

Fig. 14. Basiliximab.

### 5.4 hEN101

A novel drug hEN101 (Monarsen®; Fig. 15) is now undergoing the clinical trials. It is a representative of so called "antisense therapy", where an artificial strand of nucleic acid is designed and prepared to be complementary to mRNA, which transcript is known to be the cause of a disease (Soreq 2006). Binding of this artificial oligonucleotide to mRNA then forms an mRNA-antisense complex, which is destroyed by RNAses and the protein coded by mRNA is consequently not synthesized (Sussman 2008).

In the case of MG, the mRNA of AChE is the targeted structure. In the study performed by Brenner et al. on rats with experimental MG, the overexpression of so called "readthrough" transcript of AChE (AChE-R) was observed (Brenner 2003). AChE-R isoform might be responsible for the increased degradation of ACh in the experimental MG in rats. This isoform of AChE differs from principal synaptic isoform (AChE-S) in the structure of the C-terminal sequence (Grisaru 1999) and unlike AChE-S it forms soluble monomer, which is not anchored in the postsynaptic membrane (Seidman 1995). These structural differences make AChE-R also more sensitive to hEN101 treatment even though it binds to coding sequence of common to all isoforms. hEN101 is a 20-mer oligonucleotide active both orally and intravenously (Brenner 2003).

5´-CTGCCACGTTCTCCTGCACC-3´

hEN101

Fig. 15. hEN101.

## 6. Conclusion

The current treatment options, variety of drugs with different mechanisms of action and their availability, as well as the individual approach to the each patient have improved greatly the prognosis of MG. Though the well known AChEI are offering only symptomatic treatment that is not affecting the original cause of the disease, they are valuable tools for early and mild MG forms. The corticosteroid treatment may be also successfully applied in mild MG stages, especially in combination with immunosuppresants that allow the reduction of corticosteroid dosage. However, the biggest disadvantage of AChEI, corticosteroids or immunosuppresants and even their combination consist in their very serious side effects. For these reason, the upcoming (emerging) biological treatment seems to be solution for MG treatment. The use of monoclonal antibodies and fusion proteins that possess the specific targeted effect and only few side effects is the great benefit for the patients and this benefit is also compensating the high costs of this treatment. Moreover, the antisense therapy might solve some more issues connected to MG treatment.

## 7. Acknowledgements

This work was supported by the the Grant Agency of the Czech Republic (No. 203/09/P130), the Grant Agency of the Charles University (No. 117909/2009/B-CH/FaF), the Ministry of Health of the Czech Republic (No. MZO00179906) and the Ministry of Defense of the Czech Republic (No. MO0FVZ0000501).

## 8. References

Aeschlimann, J. A. (1933) Disubstituted carbamic acid esters of phenols containing a basic constituent. US patent US1905990

Alsberg, C. L.; Black, O. F. (1912) USDA Bur. Plant Ind. Bull., Vol.270, pp. 7

Amlot, P.L.; Akbar, A. N.; Heinrich, G.; Cammisuli, S. (1991) CD 25 binding molecules. European patent EP0449769

Anderson, D. R.; Rastetter, W. H.; Hanna, N.; Leonard, J. E.; Newman, R. A.; Reff, M. E. (1994) Therapeutic application of chimeric and radiolabeled antibodies to human B lymphocyte restricted differentiation antigen for treatment of B cell lymphoma. patent WO9411026

Anderson, D. R.; Hanna, N.; Leonard, J. E.; Newman, R. A.; Reff, M. E.; Rastetter, W. H. (1998) Therapeutic application of chimeric and radiolabeled antibodies to human B lymphocyte restricted differentiation antigen for treatment of B cell lymphoma. US patent US5776456

Arnold, H.; Bourseaux, F. (1958) Synthese und abbau cytostatisch wirksamer cyclisher N-Phosphamid ester des his (R-chlorethyl-) amins. *Angewandte Chemie*, Vol.70, No. 17, pp. 539, ISSN 1433-7851

Braun, S.; Askanas, V.; Engel, W.K.; Ibrahim, E.N. (1993). Long-term treatment with glucocorticoids increases synthesis and stability of junctional acetylcholine receptors on innervated cultured human muscle. *Journal of Neurochemistry*, Vol.60, No.5, pp. 17-20, ISSN 0022-3042

Brenner, T.; Hamra-Amitay, Y.; Evron, T. et al. (2003). The role of readthrough acetylcholinesterase in the pathophysiology of myasthenia gravis. *FASEB Journal*, Vol.17, No.2, pp. 214–222, ISSN 0892-6638

Chaudhry, V.; Cornblath, D.R.; Griffin, J.W.; O'Brien, R.; Drachman, D.B.; (2001). Mycophenolate mofetil: a safe and promising immunosuppressant in neuromuscular diseases. *Neurology*, Vol.56, No.1, pp. 94–96, ISSN 0893-0341

Ciafaloni, E.; Massey, J.M.; Tucker-Lipscomb, B.; Sanders, D.B. (2001). Mycophenolate mofetil for myasthenia gravis: an open-label pilot study. *Neurology*, Vol.56, No.1, pp. 97–99, ISSN 0893-0341

Cohn, R.G.; Mirkovich, A.; Dunlap, B.; Burton, P.; Chiu, S.H.; Eugui, E.; Caulfield, J.P. (1999). Mycophenolic acid increases apoptosis, lysosomes and lipid droplets in human lymphoid and monocytic cell lines. *Transplantation*, Vol.68, No.3, pp. 411–418, ISSN 1534-0608

Conejo-Garcia, A.; Pisani, L.; Nunez, Mdel. C.; Catto, M.; Nicolotti, O.; Leonetti, F.; Campos, J.M.; Gallo, M.A.; Espinosa, A.; Carotti, A. (2011) Homodimeric bis-quaternary heterocyclic ammonium salts as potent acetyl- and butyrylcholinesterase inhibitors: a systematic investigation of the influence of linker and cationic heads over affinity and selectivity. *Journal of Medicinal Chemistry*, Vol.54, No.8, pp. 2627-2645, ISSN 0022-2623

De Feo, L.G.; Schottlender, J.; Martelli, N.A.; Molfino, N.A. (2002) Use of intravenous pulsed cyclophosphamide in severe, generalized myasthenia gravis. *Muscle Nerve*, Vol.26, No.1, pp. 31–36, ISSN 1097-4598

Duddridge, M.; Powell, R.J. (1997). Treatment of severe and difficult cases of systemic lupus erythematosus with tacrolimus. A report of free cases. *Annals of the Rheumatic Diseases*, Vol.56, No.11, pp.690-692, ISSN 0003-4967

Durez, P.; Appelboom, T.; Pira, C.; Stordeur, P.; Vray, B.; Goldman, M. (1999). Antiinflammatory properties of mycophenolate mofetil in murine endotoxemia: inhibition of TNF-alpha and upregulation of IL-10 release. *International Journal of Immunopharmacology*, Vol.21, No.9, pp. 581–587, ISSN 0192-0561

Eisenberg, R.; Looney, R.J. (2005). The terapeutic potential of anti-CD20. "What do B cells do?" *Clinical Immunology,* Vol.117, No.3, pp. 207–213, ISSN 1521-6616

Eugui, E.M.; Mirkovich, A.; Allison, A.C. (1991). Lymphocyte-selective antiproliferative and immunosuppressive activity of mycophenolic acid and its morpholinoethyl ester (RS-61443) in rodents. *Transplantation Proceedings,* Vol.23, No.2, pp. 15–18, ISSN 0041-1345

Gajdos, P.; Elkharrat, D.; Chevret, S. et al. (1983). Arandomised clinical trial comparing prednisone and azathioprine in myasthenia gravis of the second interim analysis. *Journal of Neurology Neurosurgery and Psychiatry,* Vol.56, No.11, pp. 1157-1163, ISSN 00223050

Garcia-Carrasco, M.; Escarcega, R.O.; Fuentes-Alexandro, S.; Riebeling, C.; Cervera, R. (2007). Therapeutic options in autoimmune myasthenia gravis. *Autoimmunity reviews,* Vol.6, No.6, pp. 373-378, ISSN 1568-9972

Gremillion, R.B.; Posever, J.O.; Manek, N.; West, J.P.; van Volen-Hoven, RF. (1999) Tacrolimus (FK506) in the treatment of severe, refraktory rheumatoid arthritis: initial experience in 12 patients. *Journal of Rheumatology,* Vol.26, No.11, pp. 2332-2336, ISSN 0315-162X

Grisaru, D.; Sternfeld, M.; Eldor, A. et al. (1999). Structural roles of acetylcholinesterase variants in biology and pathology. *European Journal of Biochemistry,* Vol.264, No.3, pp. 672–686, ISSN 0014-2956

Hassan, M. M.; Al-Yahya, M. A. (1987), *Analytical Profiles of Drug Substances,* Vol.16, No.1, pp. 145-206, ISSN 1075-6280

Hauser, R.A.; Malek, A.R.; Rosen, R. (1998). Successful treatment of a patient with severe refractory myasthenia gravis using mycophenolate mofetil. *Neurology,* Vol.51, No.3, pp. 912–913, ISSN 0893-0341

Haward, C.W.H.; Fonsea, V. (1990). New treatment approaches to myasthenia gravis. *Drugs,* Vol.39, No.1, pp. 66-73, ISSN 0012-6667

Herrllinger, U.; Weller, M.; Dichgans, J.; Melms, A. (2000). Association of primary central nervous system lymphoma with long-term azathioprine therapy for myasthenia gravis. *Annals of Neurology,* Vol.47, No.5, pp. 682-683, ISSN 0364-5134

Hill, M. (2003). The neuromuscular junction disorders. *Journal of Neurology, Neurosurgery and Psychiatry,* Vol.74, No.2, pp. 32–37, ISSN 0022-3050

Hitchings, G. H.; Elion, G. B. (1962) Purine derivatives. US patent US3056785

Hodge, A.S.; Humphrey, D.R.; Rosenberry, T.L. (1992). Ambenonium is a rapidly reversible noncovalent inhibitor of acetylcholinesterase, with one of the highest known affinities. *Molecular Pharmacology,* Vol.41, No.5, pp. 937-942, ISSN 0026-895X

Hohlfeld, R.; Michels, M.; Heininger, K.; Besinger, U.; Toyka, K.V. (1988). Azathioprine toxicity during long-term immunosuppression of generalized myasthenia gravis. *Neurology,* Vol.38, No.2, pp. 258-261, ISSN 0893-0341

Hojo, M.; Morimoto, T.; Maluccio, M.; Asano, T.; Morimoto, K.; Lagman, M. et al. (1999). Cyclosporine induced cancer progression by a cell-autonomous mechanism. *Nature,* Vol.397, No.6719, pp. 530–534, ISSN 0028-0836

Jacobs, C. A.; Smith, C. A. (1997) Methods of lowering active TNF-α levels in mammals using tumor necrosis factor receptor. US patent US5605690

Juel, V.C.; Massey, J.M. (2005). Autoimmune myasthenia gravis: recommendations for treatment and immunologic modulation. *Current Treatment Options in Neurology*, Vol.7, No.1, pp. 3–14, ISSN 1534-3138

Juel, V.C.; Massey, J.M. (2007) Myasthenia gravis. *Orphanet Journal of Rare Diseases*, Vol.2, No.1, pp. 44, ISSN 1750-1172

Kahan, B.D. (1989). Cyclosporine. *New England Journal of Medicine*, Vol.321, No.25, pp. 1725-1737, ISSN 0028-4793

Kakoulidou, M.; Pirskanenn-Matell, R.; Lefvert, A.K. (2008) Treatment of a patient with myasthenia gravis using antibodies against CD25. *Acta Neurologica Scandinavica* Vol.117, No.3, pp. 211–216, ISSN 1600-0404

Kawaguchi, N. (2007). Tacrolimus treatment in Myasthenia gravis. *Current Drug Therapy*, Vol.2, No.1, pp.53-56, ISSN 1574-8855

Kino, T.; Hatanaka, H.; Hashimoto, M. et al. (1987). FK-506, a novel immunosuppressant isolated from a Streptomyces. I. Fermentation, isolation, and physico-chemical and biological characteristics. *Journal of Antibiotics*, Vol.40, No.9, pp. 1249-1255, ISSN 0021-8820

Kirchner, F. K. (1958) German patent DE1024517

Kissel, J.T.; Levy, R.J.; Mendell, J.R.; Griggs, R.C. (1986). Azathioprine toxicity in neuromuscular disease. *Neurology*, Vol.36, No.1, pp. 35-39, ISSN 0893-0341

Kokontis, L.; Gutmann, L. (2000). Current treatment of neuromuscular diseases. *Archives of Neurology*, Vol.57, No.7, pp. 939–943, ISSN 0003-9942

Komloova, M.; Musilek, K.; Dolezal, M.; Gunn-Moore, F.; Kuca, K. (2010) Structure-activity relationship of quaternary acetylcholinesterase inhibitors - Outlook for early Myasthenia gravis treatment. *Current Medicinal Chemistry*, Vol.17, No.17, pp. 1810-1824, ISSN 0929-8673

Komloova, M.; Musilek, K.; Horova, A.; Holas, O.; Dohnal, V.; Gunn-Moore, F.; Kuca, K. (2011) Preparation, in vitro screening and molecular modelling of symmetrical bisquinolinium cholinesterase inhibitors - implications for early Myasthenia gravis treatment. *Bioorganic & Medicinal Chemistry Letters*, Vol.21, No.8, pp. 2505-2509, ISSN 0960-894X

Leonetti, F.; Catto, M.; Nicolotti, O.; Pisani, L.; Cappa, A.; Stefanachi, A.; Carotti A. (2008) Homo- and hetero-bivalent edrophonium-like ammonium salts as highly potent, dual binding site AChE inhibitors. *Bioorganic & Medicinal Chemistry*, Vol.16, No.15, pp. 7450-7456, ISSN 0968-0896

Mantegazza, R.; Antozzi, C.; Peluchetti, D. (1988). Azathioprin as a single drug or in combination with steroids in the treatment of myasthenia gravis. *Journal of Neurology*, Vol.235, No.8, pp. 449-453, ISSN 0340-5354

Matsuda, S.; Koyasu, S. (2000). Mechanism of action of cyclosporine. *Immunopharmacology*, Vol.47, No.2-3, pp. 119–125, ISSN 0162-3109

Mayer, A.D.; Dmitrewski, J.; Squifflet, J-P et al. (1997) Multicenter randomized trial comparing tacrolimus (FK506) and cyclosporine in the prevention of renal allograft rejection: a report of the European Tacrolimus Multicenter Renal Study Group. *Tranplantation*, Vol. 64, No.3, pp. 436-443, ISSN 1534-0608

Meriggioli, M.N.; Rowin, J.; Richman, J.G.; Leurgans, S. (2003). Mycophenolate mofetil for myasthenia gravis: a double-blind, placebo-controlled pilot study. *Annals of the New York Academy of Sciences*, Vol.998, No.1, pp. 494–499, ISSN 0077-8923

Musilek, K.; Komloova, M.; Zavadova, V.; Holas, O.; Hrabinova, M.; Pohanka, M.; Dohnal, V.; Nachon, F.; Dolezal, M.; Kuca, K.; Jung, Y.-S. (2010) Preparation and in vitro screening of symmetrical bispyridinium cholinesterase inhibitors bearing different connecting linkage – initial study for Myasthenia gravis implications. *Bioorganic & Medicinal Chemistry Letters*, Vol.20, No.5, pp. 1763–1766, ISSN 0960-894X

Musilek, K.; Komloova, M.; Holas, O.; Hrabinova, M.; Pohanka, M.; Dohnal, V.; Nachon, F.; Dolezal, M.; Kuca, K. (2011) Preparation and in vitro screening of symmetrical bis-isoquinolinium cholinesterase inhibitors bearing various connecting linkage – implications for early Myasthenia gravis treatment. *European Journal of Medicinal Chemistry*, Vol. 6, No.2, pp. 811-818, ISSN 0223-5234

Nevins, T.E. (2000). Overview of new immunosuppressive therapy. *Current Opinion in Pediatrics*, Vol.12, No.2, pp. 146-150, ISSN 10408703

Nyberg-Hnasen, R.; Gjerstad, L. (1988). Sandimun in the treatment of myasthenia gravis. *Acta Neurologica Scandinavica*, Vol.77, No.4, pp. 307-313, ISSN 1600-0404

Okuhara, M.; Tanaka, H.; Goto, T.; Kino, T.; Hatanaka, H. (1986) Tricyclo compounds, a process for their production and a pharmaceutical composition containing the same. European patent EP0184162

Oliveto, E. P.; Gould, D. H. (1959) Process for the preparation of steroidal dienes and intermediates obtained thereby. US patent US2897216

Pascual, J.; Marcén, R.; Ortun~o, J. (2001). Anti-interleukin-2 receptor antibodies: basiliximab and daclizumab. *Nephrology Dialyses Transplantation*, Vol.16, No.9, pp. 1756–1760, ISSN 0931-0509

Richman, D.P.; Agius, M.A. (2003) Treatment of autoimmune myasthenia gravis. *Neurology*, Vol.61, No.12, pp. 1652–1661, ISSN 0893-0341

Rovin, J. (2008) Etanercept treatment in myasthenia gravis. *Annals of the New York Academy of Sciences*, Vol.1132, No.1, pp. 300–304, ISSN 0077-8923

Santa, T.; Engel, A.G.; Lambert, E.H. (1972). Histomeric study of neuromuscular junction ultrastructure I. Myasthenia gravis. *Neurology*, Vol.22, No.1, pp. 71-82, ISSN 0893-0341

Saperstein, D.S.; Barohn, R.J. (2004). Management of myasthenia gravis. *Seminars in Neurology*, Vol.24, No.1, pp. 41–48, ISSN 0271-8235

Schmid, O. (1957) Bis-carbamic acid ester compounds, and a process of making same. US patent US2789981

Seidman, S.; Sternfeld, M.; Aziz-Aloya R. B. et al. (1995). Synaptic and epidermal accumulations of human acetylcholinesterase are encoded by alternative 3'-terminal exons. *Molecular and Cellular Biology*, Vol.15, No.6, pp. 2993–3002, ISSN 0270-7306

Seybold, M.E.; Drachman, D.B. (1974). Gradually increasing doses of prednisone in myasthenia gravis: reducing the hazards of treatment. *New England Journal of Medicine*, Vol.290, No.2, pp. 81-84, ISSN 0028-4793

Sghirlanzoni, A.; Peluchetti, D.; Mantegazza, R.; Fiacchino, F.; Cornelio, F. (1984). Myasthenia gravis: prolonged treatment with steroids. *Neurology*, Vol.34, No.2, pp. 170-174, ISSN 0893-0341

Sghirlanzoni, A.; Pareyson, D.; Benuenuti, C. et al. (1992). Efficacy if intranasal administration of neostigmine in myasthenia patients. *Journal of Neurology*, Vol. 239, No.3, pp. 165-171, ISSN 0340-5354

Schneider-Gold, C.; Gajdos, P.; Toyka, K.V.; Hohlfeld, R.R. (2005). Corticosteroids for myasthenia gravis. *Cochrane Database of Systematic Reviews*, Vol.2, No.1, pp. CD002828, ISSN 1469-493X

Schwendimann, R.N.; Burton, E.; Minagar, A. (2005) Management of myasthenia gravis. *American Journal of Therapeutics*, Vol.12, No.3, pp. 262–268, ISSN 1075-2765

Smith, C. A.; Jacobs, C. A. (1994) A method for treating TNF-dependent inflammatory diseases in a mammal by administering a TNF antagonist, such as soluble TNFR. patent WO9406476

Sobotkova, M.; Bartunkova, J. (2008). Monoclonal antibodies and other biological drugs used in immunosuppressive therapy. *Remedia*, Vol.18, No.5, pp. 356-364, ISSN 0862-8947

Solsky, M.A.; Wallace, D.J. (2002) New therapies in systemic lupus erythematosus. *Best Practice and Research Clinical Rheumatology*, Vol.16, No.2, pp. 293-312, ISSN 1521-6942

Soreq, H.; Saidman, S.; Saidman, J.; Evron, T. (2006) Antisense oligonucleotide against human acetylcholinesterase (AChE) and uses thereof. US patent US7074915

Sussman, J.D.; Argov, Z.; McKee, D.; Hazum, E.; Brawer, S.; Soreq, H. (2008). Antisense treatment for myasthenia gravis: experience with Monarsen. *Annals of the New York Academy of Sciences*, Vol.1132, No.1, pp. 283–290, ISSN 0077-8923

Thanvi, B.R.; Lo, T.C.N. (2004) Update on myasthenia gravis. *Postgraduate Medical Journal*, Vol.80, No.950, pp. 690-700, ISSN 0032-5473.

Tindall, R.S.; Phillips J.T.; Rollins J.A.; Wells L.; Hall K. (1993) A clinical therapeutic trial of cyclosporine in myasthenia gravis. *Annals of the New York Acadamy of Sciences*, Vol.681, No.1, pp. 539–551, ISSN 0077-8923

Urban, R. (1951) Disubstituted carbamic acid esters of 3-hydroxy-1-alkyl-pyridinium salts. US patent US2572579

Verma, P.; Orger, J. (1992). Treatment of acquired autoimmune myasthenia gravis: a topic review. *Canadian Journal of Neurological Sciences*, Vol.19, No.3, pp. 360-375, ISSN 0317-1671

Vincenti, F. (2001). Tacrolimus (FK 506) in kidney transplantation: fiveyear survival results of the U.S. multicenter, randomized, komparative trial. *Transplantation Proceedings*, Vol.33, No.1-2, pp. 1019-1020, ISSN 0041-1345

Yang-Min, N.; Edwin, R.S. (1993) Potentiation of glucocorticoid receptormediated gene expression by the immunophilin ligands FK506 and rapamycin. *Journal of Biological Chemistry*, Vol.268, No.9, pp. 6073-6076, ISSN 0021-9258

Yazici, Y.; Abrahamson, S.B. (2007) Rheumatoid artritis treatment and monitoring of outcomes - Where are we in 2007? Controversies and opportunities. *Bulletin of the NYU Hospital for Joint Diseases,* Vol.65, No.4, pp. 300–305, ISSN 0018-5647

Zhu, L.P.; Cupps, T.R.; Whalen, G.; Fauci, A.S. (1987). Selective effects of cyclophosphamide therapy on activation, proliferation, and differentiation of human B-cells. *Journal of Clinical Investigation,* Vol.79, No.4, pp. 1082–1090, ISSN 0021-9738

# 4

# Immunomodulatory Treatments for Myasthenia Gravis: Plasma Exchange, Intravenous Immunoglobulins and Semiselective Immunoadsorption

Fulvio Baggi and Carlo Antozzi
*Neuroimmunology and Muscle Pathology Unit*
*Neurological Institute Foundation "Carlo Besta", Milan*
*Italy*

## 1. Introduction

Myasthenia Gravis (MG) is an autoimmune disorder characterized clinically by fluctuating muscle weakness and fatigability on exertion. The disease is caused by specific autoantibodies against proteins of the neuromuscular junction (NMJ) (Conti-Fine et al, 2002; Sanders & Meriggioli, 2009). Two different autoantibodies are routinely detectable, i.e. antibodies against the acetylcholine receptor (AChR) or to a muscle specific tyrosine kinase (MuSK) (Hoch et al., 2001). Anti acetylcholine receptor autoantibodies are detected in about 80-85% of patients with generalized Myasthenia Gravis. Myasthenia Gravis patients without antibodies to either acetylcholine receptor or MuSK are now defined as affected with "seronegative Myasthenia Gravis". A recent study reported that a proportion of seronegative patients has low-affinity antibodies to acetylcholine receptor, antibodies that cannot be detected by common radioimmunoassay (Leite et al., 2008).

In Myasthenia Gravis associated with anti-acetylcholine receptor antibodies the neuromuscular transmission is impaired because of the reduced number of functional acetylcholine receptors. At least three antibody-mediated mechanisms have been described to explain acetylcholine receptor impairment: accelerated endocytosis and degradation of acetylcholine receptor, functional blockade of acetylcholine-binding sites and complement-mediated damage of the post-synaptic membrane (Conti-Fine et al., 2002). The pathogenicity of anti-muscle specific tyrosine kinase antibodies is still a matter of investigation (Guptill & Sanders, 2010).

Anti-muscle specific tyrosine kinase antibodies belong to the Immunoglobulin-4 subclass of immunoglobulins and do not bind complement. Muscle specific tyrosine kinase is necessary for the agrin-mediated clustering of acetylcholine receptors on the surface of the postsynaptic membrane. It has been shown that passive transfer of immunoglobulins from anti-muscle specific tyrosine kinase positive patients can cause myasthenia when injected into mice; moreover, acetylcholine receptor density was reduced and a loss of the normal apposition between the presynaptic and postsynaptic structures has been reported (Cole et al., 2008), Therefore, apart from the above mentioned differences, anti-acetylcholine receptor and anti-muscle specific tyrosine kinase antibodies interfere with neuromuscular transmission and hence modulation of their activity can produce clinical improvement.

Myasthenia gravis is currently treated with several therapeutic approaches with the aim to induce pharmacological remission and, when possible, complete stable remission (Richman & Agius, 2003; Mantegazza et al., 2011). These approaches include: a) symptomatic treatment with anticholinesterase inhibitors, b) corticosteroids and immunosuppressive drugs to keep autoreactivity against the antigenic targets under control, and c) thymectomy, that removes surgically a potential site of autosensitization and/or perpetuation of the autoimmune process underlying the disease.

Immunomodulation in myasthenia gravis is considered a therapeutic tool able to modulate and hence interfere with the activity of specific autoantibodies. In this regard, myasthenia gravis represents a candidate disorder for the use of these treatments since, compared with other autoimmune diseases, the pathogenetic mechanisms are well characterized, and both autoantibodies and antigenic targets have been identified.

Modulation of autoantibody activity can be obtained by either their removal from plasma by means of different apheretic techniques such as therapeutic plasma exchange (TPE) or selective immunoadsorption (IA), or by expansion of the circulating immunoglobulin pool by infusion of high dose intravenous immunoglobulins (IVIG) that interfere with their activity by means of several, and still poorly understood, biological mechanisms. Removal of immunoglobulins by TPE or expansion of the total circulating pool by intravenous immunoglobulins represent opposite approaches able to induce a rapid improvement of the patients' clinical condition. Their use has been initially proposed as a form of "rescue treatment" for myasthenia gravis patients affected with the most severe forms of the disease (i.e. patients with bulbar and or respiratory involvement, patients admitted to the intensive care for respiratory insufficiency needing mechanical ventilation). Subsequently, their long-term use as been proposed for chronic immunomodulation of patients refractory to standard immunosuppression.

## 2. Therapeutic apheresis in MG

Therapeutic apheresis includes techniques able to remove different blood components. TPE is the standard procedure to separate the patient's plasma from blood cells. Plasma is obtained by means of centrifugation with computerized continuous flow cell separators or by separation with hollow fibers filters. The plasma obtained is substituted by a replacement fluid, usually 4-5% albumin solution.

The procedure is generally well tolerated; however, particular attention must be given to the patient's general clinical conditions, coagulation status and presence of cardiovascular contraindications.

Two vascular accesses are needed, the first for blood inflow, and the second one for reinfusion of blood cells mixed with the replacement fluid. A critical point is the evaluation of vascular accesses that means the availability of peripheral veins able to provide an adequate blood flow; if not, central catheters should be positioned, with higher costs and potential side effects, particularly infections when they must be left in place for several days.

A single needle approach is also feasible with some cell separators, even though more time consuming.

The use of TPE in Myasthenia Gravis was reported for the first time in 1976 (Pinching and Newsom-Davis, 1976). Since the first report, TPE has become a critical therapeutic tool for Myasthenia Gravis (Mandawat et al., 2010). Myasthenia Gravis is the best candidate disorder for treatment with TPE because of the definite role of specific autoantibodies against acetylcholine receptor or muscle specific tyrosine kinase, the two antigenic targets of the neuromuscular junction reported so far in Myasthenia Gravis.

In 1986, the National Institute of Health (NIH) held a Consensus Conference on the use of TPE in Myasthenia Gravis and concluded that TPE is effective in the short-term and that a placebo-controlled trial would not be feasible nor ethically justified (NIH, 1986; Assessment of Plasmapheresis, American Academy of Neurology 1996). Therefore, no evidence-based information is available in the literature (Cortese et al., 2011). The analysis of open studies is difficult due to their heterogeneity; indeed, exchange protocols differed among studies, treated patients were either in myasthenic crisis or prolonged worsening and the effect of ongoing treatments with steroids and disease duration are likely to have considerably influenced the results.

Methodological flaws related to these studies have been underlined in the Cochrane review on this topic (Gajdos et al., 2002). Open studies showed that TPE was effective in at least 60-70% of treated patients and that improvement was strictly related in time with plasma removal. The heterogeneity of treatment protocols in terms of number of sessions is so wide that a definite conclusion on the optimal number of sessions to be performed cannot be achieved. In some studies the number was fixed while in others patients were submitted to a number of exchange sessions apparently dependent on the achievement of a detectable clinical improvement.

In clinical practice, we adopt a conservative approach consisting of a short protocol of two exchanges performed every other day with removal of one plasma volume per session; in our hands this protocol was effective in 70% of treated patients, all affected with bulbar Myasthenia Gravis (Antozzi et al., 1991). We routinely evaluate the patient within seven days and repeat the same protocol in case of failure. We favour a conservative approach that can be effective in a short period of time instead of performing several exchanges as default. This is important considering the patient's tolerability, particularly when vascular accesses are poor. The majority of authors usually recommend three to six exchanges removing 1-1.5 plasma volumes with saline and 5% albumin replacement, performed every other day. We prefer the alternate days schedule because of the immunoglobulin backflow from the extravascular to the intravascular space.

The main indication to TPE in Myasthenia Gravis is the acute worsening of the disease (either severe generalized or bulbar) or myasthenic crisis. Other indications include worsening during the start of corticosteroids, and preparation to thymectomy in symptomatic patients. On the basis of our experience we think there is no need to perform TPE immediately before thymectomy when Myasthenia Gravis is well controlled by pharmacological treatment.

The chronic use of TPE in Myasthenia Gravis has never been addressed with a definite protocol. Nevertheless, TPE can be used at repeated intervals in selected patients in case of frequent relapses, when the response to pharmacological treatment is unsatisfactory after an adequate clinical follow-up, or in patients that have major contraindications to long-terms corticosteroids. Limitations to the use of chronic TPE are the need for good vascular accesses and the obvious effects on several plasma components in case of intensive and prolonged protocols. Therefore, the number of sessions and interval between them must be tailored on each patient taking into account the general clinical conditions, severity of Myasthenia Gravis, and potential side effects. Because of these limitations, selective apheresis should be the technique of choice in severe immunosuppression-resistant patients requiring prolonged apheretic treatments (Antozzi et al., 1994).

As mentioned earlier, antibodies to muscle specific tyrosine kinase have been reported in a proportion of patients in which anti- acetylcholine receptor antibodies were not detectable (Sanders & Meriggioli, 2009). These patients can be differentiated on clinical grounds from those with anti- acetylcholine receptor antibodies. Their clinical picture is characterized by a typical "oculo-bulbar" involvement and more frequent respiratory compromise and occurrence of myasthenic crisis requiring mechanical ventilation (Evoli et al, 2003). The disease in these patients is frequently refractory to standard immunosuppressive regimens for variable periods of time; nevertheless, muscle specific tyrosine kinase-positive Myasthenia Gravis shows a good response to TPE (or intravenous immunoglobulins) (Guptill et al., 2011). This feature is of particular importance in the effort to overcome the prolonged bulbar involvement that frequently occurs in this subset of Myasthenia Gravis patients. Treatment protocols are similar to those adopted for acetylcholine receptor-positive Myasthenia Gravis.

## 3. Semiselective immunoadsorption

The ideal apheretic approach should remove only the specific autoantibody involved in the pathogenesis of the disease under treatment, leaving all the other plasma components unaltered. Such a specific approach is not yet available for clinical practice. A compromise is represented by a technique able to remove only circulating immunoglobulins (IgGs) and hence the specific autoantibody. This technique is called semiselective immunoadsorption (IA).

Different ligands are available for clinical use in immunoglobulin-mediated disorders.

The first to be introduced was protein A (Samuelsson, 2001). Protein A is a component of the staphylococcal cell wall with the particular feature of binding human immunoglobulins with high affinity; the binding is thought to be mediated by the Fc fragment of immunoglobulins. Moreover, protein A has several other features that make it an ideal candidate for semiselective immunoadsorption: the protein has a negligible interaction with other plasma components, is stable to wide variations in temperature and pH, and can be easily regenerated.

A second method involves the use of polyclonal sheep anti-human immunoglobulins that remove directly circulating immunoglobulins by means of an immunological interaction (Nakaji 2001). In both cases, plasma must be separated by centrifugation, and is then passed on-line through a set of two filters filled with either protein A or sheep anti-human immunoglobulin. The filters are operated by dedicated monitors and work alternatively; while the first filter removes immunoglobulins, the second one is washed, submitted to the elution process to remove the adsorbed immunoglobulins, and then filled with a buffer solution, ready for the next adsorption cycle. These particular features make these techniques suitable for treatment of unlimited amounts of plasma since no replacement fluid is needed and the interaction with coagulation factors is negligible.

A different kind of semiselective immunoadsorption uses filters containing tryptophan-linked polyvinyl alcohol gel, used to treat Myasthenia Gravis patients with promising initial results in terms of clinical improvement (Grob et al., 1995; Shibuya et al., 1994). The binding is mediated by a chemical interaction and is much less selective than protein A or sheep anti-human immunoglobulin since other plasma components are retained, particularly fibrinogen and complement. A variable range of reduction of immunoglobulin and specific antibodies has been reported. The procedure does not seem to be more clinically effective than TPE and further studies should be performed to compare different methods. Moreover, these filters cannot be regenerated and therefore do not allow unlimited removal of immunoglobulins as occurs with protein A or sheep anti-human immunoglobulin.

From a technical standpoint semiselective immunoadsorption is more complicated and expensive then TPE. The procedure takes several hours since at least two plasma volumes should be treated during each session to fully exploit the binding capacity of the filters. Our treatment protocol consists of three sessions of at least two plasma volumes each, performed every other day. Again, considering the immunoglobulin backflow from the extra to the intravascular compartments we favour the alternate day regimen. Afterwards, we usually perform one maintenance session every four to six weeks; when clinical improvement between consecutive sessions remains stable and the interval between them can be increased to more than two months we usually stop semiselective immunoadsorption treatment. More intensive protocols can be performed safely if clinically needed since no replacement fluid is required and both methods do not interact with coagulation factors; in this regard, this method is particularly helpful in the treatment of patients needing oral anticoagulation.

Because of the complexity of the procedure, its duration, and costs, the indications to semiselective immunoadsorption are different from those of TPE that remains the first line apheretic option for acute exacerbations of Myasthenia Gravis. We favour the use of semiselective immunoadsorption in patients with treatment-resistant Myasthenia Gravis after adequate clinical follow-up, patients requiring frequent TPE to keep a satisfactory improvement, or patients with major contraindications to the use of high dose corticosteroids and/or other immunosuppressive drugs. In these patients, the periodic massive removal of circulating immunoglobulins can be of help in keeping symptoms under control.

A few experiences have been reported in the literature confirming the efficacy of semiselective immunoadsorption in the management of Myasthenia Gravis patients (Benny et al., 1999; Haas et al., 2002). During the last decade we submitted to semiselective immunoadsorption 19 treatment-resistant Myasthenia Gravis patients; the severity of the disease ranged from severe generalized to bulbar. Patients were periodically treated for a mean of 16 months. Improvement up to minimal manifestations or pharmacological remission was recorded in 18 out of 19. It is of interest that semiselective immunoadsorption was effective in 6 patients after failure of TPE or intravenous immunoglobulins. The mean corticosteroid reduction at the end of the treatment period was 42%.

The absence of detectable anti-acetylcholine receptor or anti muscle specific tyrosine kinase antibodies is not a contraindication to start semiselective immunoadsorption that was indeed dramatically effective in a "double-negative" patient. In this regard, the presence of low affinity antibodies in double-negative patients with Myasthenia Gravis might explain the clinical response to TPE of these patients (Leite et al., 2008).

After treatment of two plasma volumes we observed a mean 71% of total immunoglobulin and 82% reduction of specific autoantibodies (mean of 51 sessions) (Antozzi et al., 1994; Berta et al., 1994). Both immunoglobulin and anti-acetylcholine receptor antibody levels increase after treatment, but their synthesis does not seem to be increased by repeated removal; on the contrary, the time course of autoantibody recovery is consistent with immunoglobulin half-life. Moreover, as shown by Goldammer and colleagues, the synthesis of free light chains, a marker of current antibody synthesis, is not increased by semiselective immunoadsorption (Goldammer et al., 2002).

The effect of semiselective immunoadsorption, and its superiority compared with TPE, is likely related to the massive removal of immunoglobulin to an extent that cannot be achieved with standard TPE.

We also measured the potential influence of semiselective immunoadsorption on different circulating cytokines in patients affected with Myasthenia Gravis and found increased levels of Interleukin-10 and reduced levels of Interleukin-18 in post-IA plasma samples (Baggi et al., 2008). Interestingly, Interleukin-18 plays a role in the pathogenesis of experimental Myasthenia Gravis since the in vivo blockade of Interleukin-18 activity suppressed the clinical manifestations of the disease (Im et al., 2001); moreover, serum levels of Interleukin-18 were found to be increased in Myasthenia Gravis patients and clinical improvement correlated with its reduction (Jander & Stoll, 2002). Therefore, the effects of semiselective immunoadsorption on the immunological homeostasis might be wider and more complex than the mere mechanical removal of circulating antibodies, and deserve further laboratory investigations.

Research on semiselective immunoadsorption involves the investigation of new selective and specific techniques able to provide antigen-specific depletion of immunoglobulin, at least for anti-acetylcholine receptor antibodies. This approach has been investigated in vitro by means of immunoadsorbent columns carrying immobilized human acetylcholine receptor recombinant fragments. The immobilization of recombinant proteins on Sepharose beads and incubation with a seropositive Myasthenia Gravis sera resulted in a significant reduction in the concentration of specific autoantibodies in these sera (Zisimopoulou et al., 2008). Investigation on the scaling up of both production of recombinant proteins and their conjugation are needed to determine the feasibility of specific semiselective immunoadsorption in the human disease.

## 4. High dose intravenous immunoglobulins

Intravenous immunoglobulins, purified from human plasma, is a solution containing a wide range of antibodies against pathogens and antigens. Intravenous immunoglobulins were initially used in patients affected with hypogammaglobulinemia, given through the intramuscular route because of the high risk of anaphylactoid reactions. Subsequently, by means of improved purification techniques, intravenous immunoglobulins have become suitable for intravenous administration, with the advantage that larger doses can be administered in a shorter period of time.

In 1981, Imbach reported the effect of intravenous immunoglobulins in children with idiopathic thrombocytopenic purpura, with dramatic increase of platelets after intravenous immunoglobulins infusion (Imbach et al., 1981). Since that observation, the use of intravenous immunoglobulins has been extended to several neurological and non neurological autoimmune and inflammatory disorders (Elovaara et al., 2008; Donofrio et al., 2009).

The mechanism by which intravenous immunoglobulins exert their clinical effect in several autoimmune disorders is still unknown but several hypothesis have been proposed, including Fc receptor blockade of the reticuloendothelial system, modulation of the idiotypic-anti-idiotypic network, enhancement of regulatory T cells, inhibition of complement deposition, modulation of cytokines, growth factors and adhesion molecules, modulation of apoptosis and macrophages, and immune regulation of both B-cell and T-cell immune function (Ballow, 2011). The mechanism of action is likely to vary according to the disease. As far as Myasthenia Gravis is concerned, intravenous immunoglobulins might be effective particularly due to their influence on the idiotypic network and inhibition of complement deposition, according to the pathogenesis of the disease. Nevertheless, as for other autoimmune disorders, recent findings suggest an effect of intravenous immunoglobulins also on T cell immunoregulatory function (Maddur et al., 2010).

Intravenous immunoglobulins are given intravenously, the dose usually being 400 mg/kg body weight for 3-5 days. The infusion is generally well tolerated but potential adverse events must always be taken into consideration. Patients may experience anaphylaxis and anaphylactoid reactions, mild reactions including headache, fever and rash; renal failure, stroke and possible myocardial infarction have also been reported. Anaphylaxis may occur in the IgA-deficient patient. Hematological complications include hemolitic anemia and intravascular hemolysis. Thromboembolic complications have also been reported and attention should be paid to the patient's general conditions and risk factors (older age, hyperviscosity syndromes, underlying cardiovascular disorders, previous thromboembolic events). In patients at risk, high dose therapy should not be given in a short period of time, should be followed be adequate hydration, and higher daily doses should be avoided.

Several open studies on the efficacy of intravenous immunoglobulins in Myasthenia Gravis have been reported in the literature and despite the heterogeneity of patients included, clinical assessment and outcome evaluation, improvement in about 70% of treated patients has been reported. These studies are summarized in the Cochrane review devoted to this topic (Gajdos et al., 2008). A randomized placebo controlled trial reported the efficacy of intravenous immunoglobulins in worsening Myasthenia Gravis patients; the primary outcome was the Quantitative MG Score (QMG) assessed at baseline and at 14 and 28 days. Improvement was statistically significant at 14 days while the Quantitative MG Score at 28 days failed to reach statistic significance (Zinman et al., 2007).

The use of TPE in Myasthenia Gravis was first considered in comparison with intravenous immunoglobulin, that represents an alternative to TPE and share the same indications.

One randomized trial comparing the two treatments has been reported by the Myasthenia Gravis Clinical Study Group in France in 1997 (Gajdos et al., 1997). The study compared TPE and intravenous immunoglobulin in 87 patients with acute forms of the disease and concluded that intravenous immunoglobulins (400 mg/kg for 3 or 5 days) was as effective as TPE (3 sessions of 1.5 plasma volumes each). Criticism to this study included the lack of a control arm, the nonblinding of the plasmaexchange group, and the lack of stratification according to the antibody status. No significant superiority of 2 g/kg over 1 g/kg intravenous immunoglobulins was observed in the treatment of Myasthenia Gravis exacerbations (Gajdos et al., 2005).

Recently, the effect of intravenous immunoglobulins and TPE was compared by means of a randomized study including 84 patients, providing Class I evidence that intravenous immunoglobulins and TPE have compararable efficacy and are equally tolerated in patients with moderate to severe Myasthenia Gravis within two weeks of treatment (Barth et al., 2011).

Therefore, the general recommendation is that intravenous immunoglobulins are a safe and effective alternative treatment option to TPE as a short term treatment for acute exacerbation of Myasthenia Gravis. Moreover, they can be easily administered particularly when TPE is not available, or feasible due to inadequate vascular access, in patients with contraindications to extracorporeal circulation, and in children.

As already reported for TPE, also intravenous immunoglobulins have been used to prepare patients for thymectomy (Jensen & Bril, 2008). However, it is our opinion that the same considerations reported above for TPE are valid also for intravenous immunoglobulins, and that their administration before surgery should be limited to patients with Myasthenia Gravis conditions not adequately controlled by the ongoing treatment, particularly when bulbar symptoms and signs are present.

The long term use of intravenous immunoglobulins has been proposed but evidence based data supporting the efficacy of their chronic administration are lacking. However, open studies on a very limited number of patients reported improvement for up to 2 years (Achiron et al., 2000). It must be underlined that no control patients were included and that patients received concomitant immunosuppression. It is therefore opinion of the Cochrane review and of the European Task Force of the European Federation of Neurological Societies (Gajdos et al., 2008; Elovaara et al., 2009) that there is still insufficient evidence on the role of intravenous immunoglobulins in the long term management of Myasthenia Gravis.

As mentioned before for TPE, patients with anti-muscle specific tyrosine kinase antibodies show a positive response to intravenous immunoglobulins as reported in open studies on the clinical features of patients affected with this subgroup of Myasthenia Gravis (Guptill et al., 2011). Moreover, the controlled study reported by Zinman and coworkers (Zinman et al., 2007) included patients with muscle specific tyrosine kinase-associated Myasthenia Gravis; even though the results were not given for each antibody subgroup, the overall results indicate improvement also in patients without anti-acetylcholine receptor antibodies. This is particularly important for muscle specific tyrosine kinase-positive Myasthenia Gravis in case of respiratory insufficiency, when TPE is not available or not feasible.

## 5. Conclusions and future perspective

TPE, semiselective immunoadsorption and intravenous immunoglobulins represent different approaches able to modulate the activity of specific autoantibodies in Myasthenia

Gravis. TPE and intravenous immunoglobulins share the same indications, i.e. treatment of severe patients with a recent exacerbation of the disease. Even though evidence based data are rather limited (particularly for TPE), there is general agreement on the efficacy of both treatments in the acute, severe forms of the disease.

There is no evidence of the superiority of TPE versus intravenous immunoglobulins emerging from the studies reported; however, some authors favour the use of TPE as a first line approach particularly in patients with respiratory insufficiency; it is also opinion of some experts in the field that TPE is probably more rapid than intravenous immunoglobulins in promoting clinical improvement, but these observations remain personal opinions of physician with expertise in treatment of Myasthenia Gravis, opinions that should be confirmed by clinical studies.

Different considerations regard semiselective immunoadsorption, that is a more complicated, time consuming and expensive technique compared with TPE. Nevertheless, in selected, treatment-resistant patients (particularly those requiring repeated apheresis or showing no response to TPE or intravenous immunoglobulins) semiselective immunoadsorption can be of considerable help in the long-term management of the disease. The future of semiselective immunoadsorption is represented by the investigation of new ligands, as reported above on the in vitro activity of recombinant fragments of the acetylcholine receptor.

Several aspects regarding the use of TPE and intravenous immunoglobulins, as emerged from meta-analyses performed in the last ten years, need further investigation. In particular the use of immunomodulating therapies in the long-term management of Myasthenia Gravis, in combination with immunosuppressive drugs in order to reduce the burden corticosteroids as much as possible and hence reduce side effects. Protocols on the investigation of the optimal dosage should also be designed.

Recently, the subcutaneous administration of intravenous immunoglobulins has been proposed (Misbah et al., 2009); this route does not require a venous access and seems to be associated with fewer sided effects; on the other hand, frequent administrations are needed because the volumes infused intravenously cannot be given by the subcutaneous route. Studies are still preliminary and mainly performed in patients with inflammatory peripheral neuropathies, experiences that might be transferred to other autoimmune neurological disorders, including Myasthenia Gravis.

## 6. References

The utility of therapeutic plasmapheresis for neurological disorders. (1986). Natl Inst Health Consens Dev Conf Consens Statement, Vol. 6, No. 4, pp. 1-7, ISSN: 1048-566X (Print)

Assessment of plasmapheresis. Report of the Therapeutics and Technology Assessment Subcommittee of the American Academy of Neurology. (1996). Neurology, Vol. 47, No. 3, pp. 840-843, ISSN: 0028-3878 (Print)

Achiron, A., Barak, Y., Miron, S., & Sarova-Pinhas, I. (2000). Immunoglobulin treatment in refractory Myasthenia gravis. Muscle Nerve, Vol. 23, No. 4, pp. 551-555, ISSN: 0148-639X (Print)

Antozzi, C., Berta, E., Confalonieri, P., Zuffi, M., Cornelio, F., & Mantegazza, R. (1994). Protein-A immunoadsorption in immunosuppression-resistant myasthenia gravis. Lancet, Vol. 343, No. 8889, pp. 124, ISSN: 0140-6736 (Print)

Antozzi, C., Gemma, M., Regi, B., Berta, E., Confalonieri, P., Peluchetti, D., Mantegazza, R., Baggi, F., Marconi, M., Fiacchino, F., & Cornelio, F. (1991). A short plasma exchange protocol is effective in severe myasthenia gravis. J Neurol, Vol. 238, No. 2, pp. 103-107, ISSN: 0340-5354 (Print)

Baggi, F., Ubiali, F., Nava, S., Nessi, V., Andreetta, F., Rigamonti, A., Maggi, L., Mantegazza, R., & Antozzi, C. (2008). Effect of IgG immunoadsorption on serum cytokines in MG and LEMS patients. J Neuroimmunol, Vol. 201-202, No. pp. 104-110, ISSN: 0165-5728 (Print)

Ballow, M. (2011). The IgG molecule as a biological immune response modifier: mechanisms of action of intravenous immune serum globulin in autoimmune and inflammatory disorders. J Allergy Clin Immunol, Vol. 127, No. 2, pp. 315-323; quiz 324-315, ISSN: 1097-6825 (Electronic)

Barth, D., Nabavi Nouri, M., Ng, E., Nwe, P., & Bril, V. (2011). Comparison of IVIg and PLEX in patients with myasthenia gravis. Neurology, Vol. 76, No. 23, pp. 2017-2023, ISSN: 1526-632X (Electronic)

Benny, W. B., Sutton, D. M., Oger, J., Bril, V., McAteer, M. J., & Rock, G. (1999). Clinical evaluation of a staphylococcal protein A immunoadsorption system in the treatment of myasthenia gravis patients. Transfusion, Vol. 39, No. 7, pp. 682-687, ISSN: 0041-1132 (Print)

Berta, E., Confalonieri, P., Simoncini, O., Bernardi, G., Busnach, G., Mantegazza, R., Cornelio, F., & Antozzi, C. (1994). Removal of antiacetylcholine receptor antibodies by protein-A immunoadsorption in myasthenia gravis. Int J Artif Organs, Vol. 17, No. 11, pp. 603-608, ISSN: 0391-3988 (Print)

Cole, R. N., Reddel, S. W., Gervasio, O. L., & Phillips, W. D. (2008). Anti-MuSK patient antibodies disrupt the mouse neuromuscular junction. Ann Neurol, Vol. 63, No. 6, pp. 782-789, ISSN: 1531-8249 (Electronic)

Conti-Fine, B. M., Milani, M., & Kaminski, H. J. (2006). Myasthenia gravis: past, present, and future. J Clin Invest, Vol. 116, No. 11, pp. 2843-2854, ISSN: 0021-9738 (Print)

Cortese, I., Chaudhry, V., So, Y. T., Cantor, F., Cornblath, D. R., & Rae-Grant, A. (2011). Evidence-based guideline update: Plasmapheresis in neurologic disorders: report of the Therapeutics and Technology Assessment Subcommittee of the American Academy of Neurology. Neurology, Vol. 76, No. 3, pp. 294-300, ISSN: 1526-632X (Electronic)

Donofrio, P. D., Berger, A., Brannagan, T. H., 3rd, Bromberg, M. B., Howard, J. F., Latov, N., Quick, A., & Tandan, R. (2009). Consensus statement: the use of intravenous immunoglobulin in the treatment of neuromuscular conditions report of the AANEM ad hoc committee. Muscle Nerve, Vol. 40, No. 5, pp. 890-900, ISSN: 1097-4598 (Electronic)

Elovaara, I., Apostolski, S., van Doorn, P., Gilhus, N. E., Hietaharju, A., Honkaniemi, J., van Schaik, I. N., Scolding, N., Soelberg Sorensen, P., & Udd, B. (2008). EFNS guidelines for the use of intravenous immunoglobulin in treatment of neurological diseases: EFNS task force on the use of intravenous immunoglobulin in treatment of neurological diseases. Eur J Neurol, Vol. 15, No. 9, pp. 893-908, ISSN: 1468-1331 (Electronic)

Evoli, A., Tonali, P. A., Padua, L., Monaco, M. L., Scuderi, F., Batocchi, A. P., Marino, M., & Bartoccioni, E. (2003). Clinical correlates with anti-MuSK antibodies in generalized seronegative myasthenia gravis. Brain, Vol. 126, No. Pt 10, pp. 2304-2311, ISSN: 0006-8950 (Print)

Gajdos, P., Chevret, S., Clair, B., Tranchant, C., & Chastang, C. (1997). Clinical trial of plasma exchange and high-dose intravenous immunoglobulin in myasthenia gravis. Myasthenia Gravis Clinical Study Group. Ann Neurol, Vol. 41, No. 6, pp. 789-796, ISSN: 0364-5134 (Print)

Gajdos, P., Chevret, S., & Toyka, K. (2002). Plasma exchange for myasthenia gravis. Cochrane Database Syst Rev, Vol. No. 4, pp. CD002275, ISSN: 1469-493X (Electronic)

Gajdos, P., Chevret, S., & Toyka, K. (2008). Intravenous immunoglobulin for myasthenia gravis. Cochrane Database Syst Rev, Vol. No. 1, pp. CD002277, ISSN: 1469-493X (Electronic)

Gajdos, P., Tranchant, C., Clair, B., Bolgert, F., Eymard, B., Stojkovic, T., Attarian, S., & Chevret, S. (2005). Treatment of myasthenia gravis exacerbation with intravenous immunoglobulin: a randomized double-blind clinical trial. Arch Neurol, Vol. 62, No. 11, pp. 1689-1693, ISSN: 0003-9942 (Print)

Goldammer, A., Derfler, K., Herkner, K., Bradwell, A. R., Horl, W. H., & Haas, M. (2002). Influence of plasma immunoglobulin level on antibody synthesis. Blood, Vol. 100, No. 1, pp. 353-355, ISSN: 0006-4971 (Print)

Grob, D., Simpson, D., Mitsumoto, H., Hoch, B., Mokhtarian, F., Bender, A., Greenberg, M., Koo, A., & Nakayama, S. (1995). Treatment of myasthenia gravis by immunoadsorption of plasma. Neurology, Vol. 45, No. 2, pp. 338-344, ISSN: 0028-3878 (Print)

Guptill, J. T., & Sanders, D. B. (2010). Update on muscle-specific tyrosine kinase antibody positive myasthenia gravis. Curr Opin Neurol, Vol. 23, No. 5, pp. 530-535, ISSN: 1473-6551 (Electronic)

Guptill, J. T., Sanders, D. B., & Evoli, A. (2011). Anti-MuSK antibody myasthenia gravis: clinical findings and response to treatment in two large cohorts. Muscle Nerve, Vol. 44, No. 1, pp. 36-40, ISSN: 1097-4598 (Electronic)

Haas, M., Mayr, N., Zeitlhofer, J., Goldammer, A., & Derfler, K. (2002). Long-term treatment of myasthenia gravis with immunoadsorption. J Clin Apher, Vol. 17, No. 2, pp. 84-87, ISSN: 0733-2459 (Print)

Hoch, W., McConville, J., Helms, S., Newsom-Davis, J., Melms, A., & Vincent, A. (2001). Auto-antibodies to the receptor tyrosine kinase MuSK in patients with myasthenia gravis without acetylcholine receptor antibodies. Nat Med, Vol. 7, No. 3, pp. 365-368, ISSN: 1078-8956 (Print)

Im, S. H., Barchan, D., Maiti, P. K., Raveh, L., Souroujon, M. C., & Fuchs, S. (2001). Suppression of experimental myasthenia gravis, a B cell-mediated autoimmune disease, by blockade of IL-18. FASEB J, Vol. 15, No. 12, pp. 2140-2148, ISSN: 1530-6860 (Electronic)

Imbach, P., Barandun, S., d'Apuzzo, V., Baumgartner, C., Hirt, A., Morell, A., Rossi, E., Schoni, M., Vest, M., & Wagner, H. P. (1981). High-dose intravenous gammaglobulin for idiopathic thrombocytopenic purpura in childhood. Lancet, Vol. 1, No. 8232, pp. 1228-1231, ISSN: 0140-6736 (Print)

Jander, S., & Stoll, G. (2002). Increased serum levels of the interferon-gamma-inducing cytokine interleukin-18 in myasthenia gravis. Neurology, Vol. 59, No. 2, pp. 287-289, ISSN: 0028-3878 (Print)

Jensen, P., & Bril, V. (2008). A comparison of the effectiveness of intravenous immunoglobulin and plasma exchange as preoperative therapy of myasthenia gravis. J Clin Neuromuscul Dis, Vol. 9, No. 3, pp. 352-355, ISSN: 1537-1611 (Electronic)

Leite, M. I., Jacob, S., Viegas, S., Cossins, J., Clover, L., Morgan, B. P., Beeson, D., Willcox, N., & Vincent, A. (2008). IgG1 antibodies to acetylcholine receptors in 'seronegative' myasthenia gravis. Brain, Vol. 131, No. Pt 7, pp. 1940-1952, ISSN: 1460-2156 (Electronic)

Maddur, M. S., Othy, S., Hegde, P., Vani, J., Lacroix-Desmazes, S., Bayry, J., & Kaveri, S. V. (2010). Immunomodulation by intravenous immunoglobulin: role of regulatory T cells. J Clin Immunol, Vol. 30 Suppl 1, No. pp. S4-8, ISSN: 1573-2592 (Electronic)

Mandawat, A., Kaminski, H. J., Cutter, G., Katirji, B., & Alshekhlee, A. (2010). Comparative analysis of therapeutic options used for myasthenia gravis. Ann Neurol, Vol. 68, No. 6, pp. 797-805, ISSN: 1531-8249 (Electronic)

Mantegazza, R., Bonanno, S., Camera, G., & Antozzi, C. (2011). Current and emerging therapies for the treatment of myasthenia gravis. Neuropsychiatr Dis Treat, Vol. 7, No. pp. 151-160, ISSN: 1178-2021 (Electronic)

Meriggioli, M. N., & Sanders, D. B. (2009). Autoimmune myasthenia gravis: emerging clinical and biological heterogeneity. Lancet Neurol, Vol. 8, No. 5, pp. 475-490, ISSN: 1474-4422 (Print)

Misbah, S., Sturzenegger, M. H., Borte, M., Shapiro, R. S., Wasserman, R. L., Berger, M., & Ochs, H. D. (2009). Subcutaneous immunoglobulin: opportunities and outlook. Clin Exp Immunol, Vol. 158 Suppl 1, No. pp. 51-59, ISSN: 1365-2249 (Electronic)

Nakaji, S. (2001). Current topics on immunoadsorption therapy. Ther Apher, Vol. 5, No. 4, pp. 301-305, ISSN: 1091-6660 (Print)

Pinching, A. J., & Peters, D. K. (1976). Remission of myasthenia gravis following plasma-exchange. Lancet, Vol. 2, No. 8000, pp. 1373-1376, ISSN: 0140-6736 (Print)

Richman, D. P., & Agius, M. A. (2003). Treatment of autoimmune myasthenia gravis. Neurology, Vol. 61, No. 12, pp. 1652-1661, ISSN: 1526-632X (Electronic)

Samuelsson, G. (2001). Extracorporeal immunoadsorption with protein A: technical aspects and clinical results. J Clin Apher, Vol. 16, No. 1, pp. 49-52, ISSN: 0733-2459 (Print)

Shibuya, N., Sato, T., Osame, M., Takegami, T., Doi, S., & Kawanami, S. (1994). Immunoadsorption therapy for myasthenia gravis. J Neurol Neurosurg Psychiatry, Vol. 57, No. 5, pp. 578-581, ISSN: 0022-3050 (Print)

Zinman, L., Ng, E., & Bril, V. (2007). IV immunoglobulin in patients with myasthenia gravis: a randomized controlled trial. Neurology, Vol. 68, No. 11, pp. 837-841, ISSN: 1526-632X (Electronic)

Zisimopoulou, P., Lagoumintzis, G., Kostelidou, K., Bitzopoulou, K., Kordas, G., Trakas, N., Poulas, K., & Tzartos, S. J. (2008). Towards antigen-specific apheresis of pathogenic autoantibodies as a further step in the treatment of myasthenia gravis by plasmapheresis. J Neuroimmunol, Vol. 201-202, No. pp. 95-103, ISSN: 0165-5728 (Print)

# 5

# Respiratory Care for Myasthenic Crisis

Ping-Hung Kuo and Pi-Chuan Fan
*National Taiwan University*
*Hospital Taiwan*
*Taiwan*

## 1. Introduction

Myasthenic crisis is a life-threatening complication of myasthenia gravis (MG) that is traditionally defined as weakness of respiratory muscles that is severe enough to require intubation or artificial respiratory support (Jaretzki et al., 2000). Rapid and marked increase in limb and bulbar weakness without respiratory failure, however, should probably be also defined as crisis in a myasthenic patient. Although it is potentially life-threatening, the mortality rate has declined dramatically with better and more aggressive care in the intensive care unit (ICU) and the widespread use of immunotherapies (Varelas et al., 2002; Thomas et al., 1997). Respiratory management of these patients, however, is very challenging due to the fluctuating nature of the disease. Assiduous attention to respiratory care provides support of the patient, allowing time for therapy of the underlying myasthenia to be effective. There are deficiencies in current services for myasthenic crisis in that the ICU physicians not being expert respiratory specialists, and physicians managing mechanical ventilation not experienced in neurologic aspects of these patients.

This chapter reviews the respiratory dysfunction in myasthenic crisis and discusses issues related to respiratory care in these patients, including airway management, mechanical ventilation and extubation outcome.

## 2. Epidemiology

Myasthenic crisis occurs in 15 to 20% of patients with MG during their lifetime (Phillips, 2004 ). It usually occurs during the course of first symptomatic presentation in the young and later in the course of the disease in the elderly. The median time to first myasthenic crisis from onset of MG ranges from 8 to 12 months (Thomas et al., 1997; Rabinstein et al., 2005). However, crisis may be the initial presentation of MG in one-fifth of patients (Rabinstein et al., 2005;. O'Riordan et al., 1998). Overall, women are twice as likely as men to be affected. There is a bimodal distribution of myasthenic crisis, with an early peak prior to age 55 affecting women 4:1, whereas a later peak after age 55 affecting women and men equally (Thomas et al., 1997). The average age of admission with crisis is 59 years (Wendell et al., 2011). Pregnancy is associated with an aggravation of myasthenia gravis in approximately a third of all women and myasthenic crisis in pregnancy carries high perinatal mortality (Plauche, 1991).

The incidence of crisis remains stable from 1960s to 1990s (Cohen and Younger, 1981). Recently, an increasing incidence of MG, especially in the elderly population, has been observed in some countries (Pakzad, 2011), and the incidence of anti-acetylcholine receptor (AChR) seropositivity in the ≥ 65 age group has increased at a significantly greater rate than the rate of increase in the younger people. It is very rare for patients with myasthenia to need long-term invasive or noninvasive ventilator support, although that need is slightly more common in patients with muscle specific tyrosine kinase (MuSK) antibodies (MuSK-MG) as opposed to AChR antibodies (AChR-MG).

## 3. Precipitants of myasthenic crisis

Myasthenic crisis may be precipitated by a variety of factors, most often a concurrent infection (Mayer, 1997; Wendell and Levine, 2011′ Thomas et al., 1997). Although patients with MG can develop any common infection that can result in decompensation, the most likely source of infection is pulmonary. One series documented infection in 38% of patients presenting with myasthenic crisis. The most common cause was bacterial pneumonia, followed by a bacterial or viral upper respiratory infection (Thomas et al., 1997). Other precipitants can be surgery, menstruation, pregnancy, childbirth, or tapering of immunosuppressive medications, exposure to temperature extremes, pain, sleep deprivation, and physical or emotional stress. The precipitant may not be found in up to one-third of cases (Mayer, 1997; Thomas et al., 1997; O'Riordan et al., 1998). In addition, crisis can occur spontaneously as part of the natural history of MG itself (Thomas et al., 1997; O'Riordan et al., 1998; Juel, 2004). A number of drugs can increase the weakness in myasthenia and should be considered as possible precipitants in this setting. This is of more concern with certain antibiotics (aminoglycosides, erythromycin and azithromycin), cardiac drugs (β-blockers, procainamide, and quinidine), and magnesium (Wendell and Levine, 2011). Although corticosteroids can be used in the treatment of MG, initial treatment with prednisone led to an exacerbation of MG in almost half of patients in 1 series (Pascuzzi et al., 1984). The incidence of myasthenic crisis resulting from corticosteroids ranges from 9 to 18% (Pascuzzi et al.,1984; Bae et al., 2006). Therefore, initiation of corticosteroid therapy for the treatment of MG should always occur in a hospital setting, where respiratory function can be monitored (Pascuzzi et al, 1984). Predictors of exacerbation from prednisone include older age, lower score on the Myasthenia Severity Scale, and bulbar symptoms (Bae et al., 2006).

## 4. Pathophysiology and clinical presentations

The respiratory failure in myasthenic crisis can be of either the hypoxemic or the hypercapnic form, and may result from the combination of poor airway protection, inadequate secretion clearance and hypoventilation (Juel, 2004; Borel et al., 1993; Mier-Jedrzejowicz et al., 1988). Muscle weakness in AchR-MG tends to initially affect the intercostal and accessory muscles and then the diaphragm (Chaudhuri and Behan, 2009). Bulbar (oropharyngeal) muscle dysfunction may be the predominant feature in some patients (Putman and Wise, 1996). In MuSK-MG, bulbar weakness always precedes respiratory failure (Chaudhuri and Behan, 2009). The central ventilatory drive in myasthenics usually remains intact during crisis, even when the minute ventilation response to $CO_2$ is poor (Rabinstein and Wijdicks, 2003).

Clinically, ptosis, ophthalmoparesis, and facial and bulbar weakness are common, in addition to generalized weakness. At the bedside, recruitment of accessory muscles indicates significant inspiratory muscle weakness, and a weak cough or difficulty in counting to 20 in a single breath signifies weakness of the expiratory muscles (Juel, 2004). Patient anxiety, accompanied by tachycardia and tachypnea, may be the first sign of air hunger (Table 1). Signs of bulbar weakness include dysphagia, nasal regurgitation, a nasal quality to speech, staccato speech, jaw weakness (jaw closure weaker than jaw opening), bifacial paresis, and tongue weakness (Garcia-Pachon et al., 1996; Rabinstein and Wijdicks, 2003). The most important dysfunction of the upper airway leading to respiratory failure is laryngeal muscle weakness causing abnormal adduction of the vocal cords during inspiration and even paralysis (Friedman and Goffin, 1966). Respiratory failure may develop due to aspiration, catastrophic airway compromise, or increased work of already fatigued respiratory muscles against a closed airway (Putman and Wand, 1996).

One particular danger in myasthenic crisis is that the generalized weakness can mask the usual signs of respiratory distress. In addition, weak respiratory muscles may suddenly fatigue, producing precipitous respiratory collapse. Some patients may present with respiratory insufficiency out of proportion to limb or bulbar weakness. In rare cases of myasthenic crisis, ventilatory failure is the only clinically overt manifestation (Mier et al., 1990; Dushay et al., 1990). Therefore, signs of myasthenic crisis should be sought in all patients with MG, even when they do not complain of weakness.

| |
|---|
| Abdominal muscle paradox |
| Accessory muscle use |
| Cough after swallowing |
| Difficulty in clearing secretions |
| Dysphagia |
| Hypophonia |
| Inability to raise the head due to neck muscle weakness |
| Forehead sweating |
| Jaw weakness (jaw closure weaker than jaw opening) |
| Nasal regurgitation |
| Orthopnea |
| Pausing during speech to take a breath |
| Rapid shallow breathing |
| Staccato speech or a nasal quality to speech |
| Single breath count of < 15 |
| Stridor |
| Tachypnea |
| Tongue weakness |
| Weak cough |
| Wet, gurgling voice |

Table 1. Warning symptoms and signs of impending respiratory failure in myasthenic crisis. (Rabinstein, 2003; Bedlack and Sanders, 2002; Juel, 2004)

## 5. Assessment of respiratory muscle strength and bulbar function

### 5.1 Assessment of vital capacity (VC)

The VC reflects the mechanical function of both inspiratory and expiratory respiratory muscles and can be performed at the bedside to assess the patient's trend (Juel, 2004; Rabinstein and Wijdicks, 2003). The patient is instructed to take a deep breath in and then to exhale maximally into a spirometer. Some experts recommend assessing both supine and sitting VC, as diaphragmatic weakness is more apparent on the supine measurement. Supine VC has been shown to be an earlier marker of detect diaphragm dysfunction.

### 5.2 Assessment of inspiratory muscle function

#### 5.2.1 Maximal inspiratory pressure (PImax)

The static PImax measured during a maximal inspiratory effort that is sustained for ≥ 1 s against an occluded airway is the most widely used parameter for assessing inspiratory muscle strength, Although the early literature reported that PImax testing should be performed from residual volume (RV), more recent work has shown that it is reasonable to simplify the procedure by measuring this pressure from the functional residual capacity (FRC) (Windisch et al., 2004). The normal range of PImax values is wide and some patients may have difficulties in performing the procedure, particularly those with bulbar dysfunction.

#### 5.2.2 Sniff nasal inspiratory pressure (SNIP)

Alternative techniques have been developed over the last few years to assess the inspiratory function. One of the most promising is determination of SNIP, which consists in the measurement of pressure through an occluded nostril during sniffs, performed through the contralateral nostril (Soliman et al., 2005). The testing of SNIP should be performed from FRC. It has been shown to be a good physiological marker of inspiratory muscle strength (Martínez-Llorens et al., 2011). SNIP maneuver is easier to perform than PImax maneuver, and it is as reproducible as Pimax, However SNIP may underestimate esophageal pressure swing in subjects with nasal obstruction and severe neuromuscular weakness. Multiple tests to assess respiratory muscle strength are required to exclude weakness in symptomatic patients (Steier et al, 2007; Hart et al., 2003). Because, of the limit of agreement between SNIP and PImax, these two methods are not interchangeable but complementary (Prigent et al., 2004).

#### 5.2.3 Sensitivity of volume vs. pressure measures

It remains controversial whether volume or pressure measurements are more sensitive in the assessment of respiratory muscle function. The theoretical curvilinear relation between volume and pressure implies that, in the case of mild respiratory muscle weakness, VC is less sensitive than PImax, and, in more advanced disease, marked reduction in VC can occur with relatively small changes in maximum pressures. One previous study showed that inspiratory and expiratory forces were more sensitive than VC in evaluating muscle strength in MG (Mier-Jedrzejowicz et al., 1988). However, a recent study found that PImax was not more sensitive than VC for early detection of respiratory muscle failure in these patients (Prigent et al., 2011). Since neither measurement has been shown to be superior, the two parameters are usually analyzed in combination.

### 5.3 Assessment of expiratory muscle function

#### 5.3.1 Maximal expiratory pressure (PEmax)

The strength of the expiratory muscles can be assessed by the maximal expiratory pressure (PEmax) (Rabinstein et al., 2003), which can be measured at the mouth in an analogous fashion to PImax during a forced expiration (from total lung capacity maneuver). It represents the integration of exhalation muscle strength and sufficient cough flows have to be generated by expiratory muscles to allow airway clearance. In a study of neuromuscular diseases (Perez, 2006), PEmax below 45 cm $H_2O$ was associated with compromised cough efficiency, and PEmax < 40 cm $H_2O$ may indicate crisis (Lacomis, 2005). It is important to prevent the subject from using buccal manoeuvres to increase the mouth pressure. As with PImax, PEmax values have a wide normal range.

#### 5.3.2 Peak cough flow

Another simple and commonly used test of expiratory muscles is the peak cough flow, which can be performed using a standard peak flow meter attached to a face mask and usually requires little or no coaching to produce acceptable technique. Cough assessment is an inexact science, however, because of the lack of accurate measures. A peak cough flow value of < 270 L/min has been proposed as a threshold for cough inadequacy, but this has never been validated. Patients with a peak cough flow < 180 L/min are unable to independently clear secretions (Bach, 1995). In myasthenics, peak cough flow has been shown to be useful in monitoring expiratory muscle strength (Suárez et al., 2002; Wilson et al., 2005). It must be realized that although this test indicates expiratory muscle performance the pressure and force generated depends on lung volumes and coordinated bulbar function to rapidly open and close the glottis during cough pressure generation and release. Therefore, values obtained will be reduced in patients with inspiratory muscle weakness due to inability to perform deep inspiration prior to cough initiation (Polkey et al., 1998).

### 5.4 Assessment of bulbar function

Although critical for management decisions, reliable clinical assessment of bulbar function with MG is often difficult (Hudspeth et al., 2006). As it is well established, the involvement of upper airway muscles in neuromuscular diseases can produce abnormalities of the maximum flow-volume loop (MFVL) in the form of upper airway obstruction and/or flow oscillations (Putman and Wise, 1996). Upper airway obstruction is much more common in patients with MG than previously recognized. In one study, 7 of the 12 MG patients examined disclosed a pattern of extrathoracic upper airway obstruction (Putman and Wise, 1996). In addition, a crude but effective bedside test can be performed by asking the patient to sip water and then observing for coughing or choking. This "slurp" test has been shown to be valuable for identifying serious compromise of bulbar function and for monitoring and guiding therapy in pediatric patients with MG (Hudspeth et al., 2006).

## 6. Initial respiratory care in the ICU

The respiratory management of myasthenic crisis does not differ between patients with AChR-MG, MuSK-MG and seronegative patients (Chaudhuri and Behan, 2009).

### 6.1 Initial evaluation and airway management

Patients with crisis should be referred for intensive care. The initial step is stabilization of the airway. The airway should be opened by suctioning secretions after positioning the jaw and tongue. High-flow oxygen should be administered and oxygen saturation be monitored by pulse oximetry continuously. If respirations remain inadequate, patients can be ventilated by a bag-valve mask while preparing to intubate. In the patient without an intact gag reflex, an oral airway may be placed to prevent aspiration. Patients should always be asked about recent difficulty with swallowing, choking, coughing after eating, and nasal regurgitation. If the patient's history or the "slurp" test is suggestive of dysphagia, oral intake is eliminated.

Once the airway is secured, investigation into the cause of the exacerbation of MG may proceed. Any medication suspected of precipitating crisis should be discontinued (Keesey, 2004). Chest radiography is important in detecting pneumonia. Appropriate broad-spectrum antibiotics are indicated for sepsis and pneumonia. It is important to consider that fluoroquinolones and aminoglycosides may adversely affect muscle function in these patients, and these antibiotics should be avoided if possible.

Prompt recognition of impending respiratory paralysis is the key to successful management. The classical signs of respiratory distress, however, often occur too late in these patients to serve as guidelines for management. Respiratory assistance should be provided if VC is < 15-20 mL/kg, the tidal volume < 5–6 mL/kg, or if $PaO_2$ drops to < 85 mm Hg and $PaCO_2$ increases to > 45 mm Hg. Oxygen saturation and ABG abnormalities, however, are generally not considered ideal for use in making intubation decisions because these values change late in the decompensation cycle (Juel, 2004; Rabinstein and Wijdicks, 2003; Bird and Teener, 2001).

### 6.2 Bronchodilator therapy

One recent study found that patients with MG had significantly lower $FEV_1/FVC$ ratio than controls. This was more marked in patients on acetylcholine esterase inhibitors (Elsais et al., 2010). In myasthenic crisis, bronchodilators may be useful in maintaining airway patency and overcoming bronchospasm. For myasthenics with concomitant chronic obstructive pulmonary disease (COPD), inhaled ipratropium bromide may be the bronchodilator drug of choice because it is safe and can decreased bronchial secretions which may limit the use of cholinesterase inhibitors (Szathmáry et al., 1981; Liggett et al., 1988). A recent pilot study also suggests that terbutaline, a $\beta_2$ adrenergic agonist, may be an effective adjunct therapy in these patients, although confirmation with larger trials will be required (Soliven et al., 2011).

### 6.3 Indications and predictors for endotracheal intubation

Two-thirds to 90% of patients with myasthenic crisis require intubation and mechanical ventilation (Thomas et al., 1997; O'Riordan et al., 1998). Over 20% of patients require intubation during evaluation in the emergency department, and almost 60% are intubated after admission to an ICU (Thomas et al., 1997). The absolute indications for intubation may include cardiac or respiratory arrest, impaired consciousness shock, life-threatening arrhythmias, severe blood–gas alterations, and bulbar dysfunction with confirmed aspiration. Much more difficult is the decision to intubate when such strict criteria are not met.

In most patients, repeated measurements of VC and PImax help determine the need for and timing of elective intubation (Ahmed et al., 2005; Rabinstein and Wijdicks, 2003). These indices can be measured as often as every two hours, but typically every four hours. The standard 20/30/40 rule (VC < 20 mL/kg; PImax <_30 cm $H_2O$ and PEmax < 40 cm $H_2O$) is probably the most helpful guide to decide when intubation (Chaudhuri and Behan, 2009). However, these threshold values have not been established through prospective studies, nor do they allow for individual differences in size, sex, and age. In addition, muscle weakness in myasthenic crisis often fluctuates, and patients can develop apnea very suddenly, or may precipitously fatigue with the rapid development of respiratory failure before a downward trend in these parameters is noted. Facial weakness can also lead to inaccurate measurements of these indices due to inability to make a good seal with the mask (Lacomis, 2005). In a retrospective review, repeated measurement of VC did not predict the need for intubation and mechanical ventilation in these patients (Rieder et al., 1995). Thus, these respiratory parameters should always be interpreted in the context of the clinical symptoms and signs, as well as the trend in these measures. Regardless of respiratory function indices, the need for mechanical ventilation is a sufficient criterion to define myasthenic crisis (Ahmed et al., 2005). With close monitoring of the patient's condition, endotracheal intubation can often be performed electively rather than as an emergent response to precipitous respiratory collapse (Juel, 2004; Rabinstein and Wijdicks, 2003; Bird and Teener, 2001).

### 6.4 Procedures for endotracheal intubation

Should the need for emergent intubation develop, rapid sequence intubation should be modified because neuromuscular blocking agents (paralytics) should be used with caution when intubating these patients. Depolarizing agents (for example, succinylcholine) are less potent in myasthenics because fewer functional post-synaptic anti-AChR are available. This decrease in receptors also results in a decrease in the safety margin or remaining AChR available for neuromuscular transmission. Nondepolarizing agents (fornexample, vecuronium) have increased potency, and reduced doses are required for paralysis. (Baraka, 1992). A rapid-onset nondepolarizing agent (ie, rocuronium, vecuronium) is the preferred paralytic agent for these patients. Although nondepolarizing agents delay the onset of paralysis, compared with succinylcholine, these medications do not result in unwanted prolonged paralysis. Following paralysis, intubation is accomplished as usual. A soft, low-pressure cuff is recommended. After intubation, chest radiography should be taken to confirm the position of the artificial airway.

### 6.5 Modification of pharmacotherapy after intubation

After intubation, cholinesterase inhibitor therapy is usually temporarily withdrawn to avoid the excess secretions that may complicate pulmonary management. In addition, continued use of these medications confounds the assessment of other treatment modalities and can increase muscle weakness if used in excess (Ahmed et al., 2005). These medications do not alter the course of the crisis and offer solely symptomatic relief of MG (Juel, 2004). After patients have shown definitive improvement in muscle strength, usually several days after the initiation of intravenous immunoglobulin (IVIg) or plasma exchange, acetylcholinesterase inhibitors, typically oral pyridostigmine, can be reintroduced after or just prior to extubation (Juel, 2004; Ahmed et al., 2005). Oral pyridostigmine is preferred, but it may be given intravenously. One milligram of intravenous pyridstigmine is equal to 30 mg of oral pyridostigmine. Patients should be started on a low dose of the medication that is titrated to symptomatic relief (Ahmed et al., 2005). Continuous intravenous infusion of pyridostigmine as treatment for myasthenic crisis may have efficacy similar to that of plasma exchange, but it is associated with an increased risk of life-threatening cardiac arrhythmia (Wendell and Levine, 2011). Unless contraindicated, all patients should be treated with low molecular weight heparin to prevent deep vein thrombosis and pulmonary embolism (Chaudhuri and Behan, 2009).

## 7. Ventilatory management strategies

### 7.1 Ventilator settings

Once intubated, patients should be placed in a semi-recumbent position with the head of the bed at approximately 30 degrees. Large tidal volumes of 10 mL/kg, along with pressure support of 5 to 15 cm $H_2O$ and positive end-expiratory pressure (PEEP) of 5 to 15 cm $H_2O$, are encouraged to limit atelectasis, provided peak airway pressures can be maintained below 40 cm $H_2O$ (Kirmani et al., 2004; Varelas et al., 2002). The degree of support required is patient-dependent and should be adjusted based on ABG analysis. In patients with chronic carbon dioxide retention (suggested by elevated serum bicarbonate levels), $PaCO_2$ should be kept above 45 mm Hg to avoid alkalosis and bicarbonate wasting, which make weaning more difficult. Frequent checks of cuff pressure, tube placement, and blood gases are recommended.

### 7.2 Chest physiotherapy and airway clearance

Meticulous attention to pulmonary toilet is required because of an ineffective cough mechanism. Aggressive chest physiotherapy and airway clearance should be implemented (Varelas et al., 2002). Inspired gas humidity should be around 80% at 37°C. Various modalities, include percussion, vibration, and postural drainage. should be carried out to loosen and remove bronchial secretions and to achieve better aeration of collapsed areas of the lung (Brooks-Brunn, 1995; Lewis, 1980; Selsby and Jones, 1990). Regular suctioning serves to not only remove excess oropharyngeal and tracheal secretions but also to stimulate coughing (Varelas et al., 2002). Patients with a cough PEF < 180 L/min can augment cough response with manual physiotherapy and using insufflation-exsufflation devices (Chatwin et al., 2003) and this augmented cough level is associated with improved prognosis independent of VC or breathing pattern (Bach, 1995).

If atelectasis is severe and does not respond to routine measures, therapeutic fiberoptic bronchoscopy can be performed to promote airway toilet. Frequent body repositioning is effective in enhancing oxygen transport by changing the ventilation and perfusion of the lungs through gravitational effects and by enhancing mobilization of secretions. Early mobilization and ambulation as tolerated is also encouraged.

### 7.3 Nutrition and other issues during mechanical ventilation

Adequate nutrition is important to avoid a negative energy balance and worsening of muscle strength (Kirmani et al., 2004). All patients received adequate nutritional support (25–35 calories per kilogram) via enteral route whenever possible. In patients with hypercarbia and difficulty weaning from the ventilator, low carbohydrate feeds are the preferred solution (Varelas et al., 2002).

In addition to the aforementioned measures, abnormal laboratory values that could affect muscle strength should also be corrected. Potassium, magnesium, and phosphate depletion can all exacerbate myasthenic crisis and should be repleted. Anemia can also increase weakness, and several experts recommend transfusions when hematocrit values are under 30% (Kirmani et al., 2004; Ahmed et al., 2005). Prophylaxis for deep vein thromboses, such as administration of subcutaneous heparin sodium or use of pneumatic compression boots, is recommended.

## 8. Weaning from mechanical ventilation and risks for extubation failure

### 8.1 Disadvantages of prolonged intubation

Prolonged intubation in myasthenic patients may lead to several complications such as atelectasis, anemia, urinary tract infection, congestive heart failure (Ahmed et al., 2005), and ventilator-associated pneumonia (VAP) (Wu et al., 2008). Patients with a prolonged intubation were hospitalized 3 times longer and were less likely to be functionally independent upon discharge (Thomas et al., 1997). In one series, 3 independent risk factors for prolonged intubation (>14 days) were identified: age > 50 years, peak VC < 25 mL/kg on post-intubation days 1 to 6, and a serum bicarbonate ≥ 30 mmol/L (Thomas et al., 1997). All of the patients with no risk factors were intubated for less than 2 weeks, whereas 88% of the patients with all 3 risk factors had prolonged intubation.

### 8.2 Evaluation for weaning in myasthenia crisis

Deciding on when to stop mechanical ventilation in myasthenic crisis is a challenge for the intensivists, because the usual criteria don't necessarily apply. Evaluation for weaning should begin when patients are objectively getting stronger on examination. In addition, improvement in the strength of neck flexors and other adjunct muscles is usually associated with improvement in bulbar and respiratory muscle strength and can be a useful tool for assessing clinical improvement (Meriggioli, 2009). Patients should be transitioned to a spontaneous mode of ventilation (eg, pressure support ventilation) in which all breaths are patient initiated. Pressure support can then gradually be decreased to minimal settings, usually 5 to 8 cm $H_2O$. If results of assessments indicate muscle fatigue, the previous level of ventilator support should be reinstituted (Kirmani et al., 2004). In patients with chronic $CO_2$ retention, $PaCO_2$ should be kept above 45 mm Hg to avoid alkalosis and bicarbonate wasting, which may make weaning more difficult.

Current recommendations about managing the weaning process emphasize the daily determination of simple criteria (Fly et al., 1996; Fly et al., 1999). Some criteria are generally used: 1) Satisfactory oxygenation, for instance $PaO_2/FIO_2 \geq 200$ mm Hg with PEEP $\leq 5$ cm $H_2O$; 2) A criterion for hemodynamic stability, e.g., no continuous vasopressor infusion; 3) Patient awake or easily aroused and sedation stopped; and 4) Patient able to cough effectively.

### 8.3 Spontaneous breathing trial (SBT)

Readiness for extubation from a respiratory standpoint is largely judged on the basis of patient performance during an SBT. Two main methods are used: T-piece and a low level of

PSV, with a duration ranging from 30 min to 2 hours (Esteban et al., 1997). It should always begin early in the day. During this period, patient anxiety, pulse and respiratory rates, and tidal volume again are frequently documented. There are no good clinical criteria for when and how to try extubation safely, thus avoiding the need for reintubation. Fluctuating weakness and pulmonary complications often confound the decision to extubate (Seneviratne et al., 2008). Patients are typically extubated if VC and PImax are $\geq$ 15 mL/kg and $\leq$_- 20 cm $H_2O$, respectively, and tidal volume $\geq$ 5 mL/kg (Kirmani et al., 2004; Meriggioli, 2009). In our study, a PEmax of > 40 cm $H_2O$ was a good predictor of extubation success in these patients (Wu et al., 2009). If the patient complains of fatigue or shortness of breath, extubation should not be performed even if the criteria of these indices are met and blood gases are normal (Berrouschot et al., 1997; Gracey et al., 1983; Kelly, 1991). Our experience also indicates that the rapid shallow breathing index (breathing frequency divided by tidal volume) is a poor predictor for extubation outcome in patients with neuromuscular diseases (Kuo et al., 1996; Wu et al, 2009).

### 8.4 Potential utility of new modes of mechanical ventilation

Some new modes of mechanical ventilation, which are aimed at unloading the inspiratory muscles and preventing patient-ventilator dyssynchrony, may be useful in neuromuscular patients with difficult weaning. These modes include proportional assist ventilation (PAV), adaptive support ventilation (ASV), and neurally-adjusted ventilatory assist (NAVA). However, there is still no evidence from randomized controlled trials to support or refute the use of these modes in myasthenic crisis. Automatic tube compensation (ATC) is a special mode of ventilatory support which delivers the amount of pressure necessary to overcome the resistive load imposed by the endotracheal tube for the flow measured at the time (Fabry et al., 1994). This mode therefore unloads the flow-resistive properties of the artificial airway and can increase the probability of successful extubation. One recent report indicates that the addition of ATC to a standard PSV-based **weaning** protocol significantly shortened time needed to wean patients with severe neuromuscular paralysis (Agarwal et al., 2009). It is possible that ATC will be a useful weaning mode in myasthenic crisis, especially for patients who are intubated with a small-size endotrachel tube.

### 8.5 Respiratory care after extubation

To enhance mucous clearance and prevent sputum impaction after extubation, it is reasonable to consider airway clearance techniques, such as positive expiratory pressure, autogenic drainage, and active cycle of breathing techniques in these patients (Hardy and Anderson, 1996). The addition of mechanical insufflation/exsufflation may shorten airway-clearance sessions in neuromuscular patients with chest infection (Chatwin and Simonds, 2009). The intrapulmonary percussive ventilator and high-frequency chest wall oscillator with vests may show growing promise in this area (Toussaint et al., 2003). However, these modalities have not been specifically in myasthenics. Externally applied pressure, such as with the In-Exsufflator or the cyclically inflated pneumatic belt, can augment the patient's own efforts and is sometimes helpful. Normalizing the VC and FRC typically helps to improve the ability to cough and clear secretions. Sputum mobilization can be facilitated with the Flutter valve therapy without the assistance of another caregiver, as long as the patient has the motivation. Incentive spirometry can also be used to reduce the risk of atelectasis and re-intubation (American Association for Respiratory Care, 1991), but its usefulness in myasthenic crisis patients is not clear.

The risk of spontaneous relapse of myasthenic crisis is low in early-onset disease. A third of late onset severe disease, especially in MuSK-MG, may experience recurrent crisis (Chaudhuri and Behan, 2009). Therefore, close observation for 72 hours in the ICU is recommended for each patients after extubation. The duration of observation may have to be longer for less stable patients.

### 8.6 Extubation outcome and the risk of extubation failure

The rate of extubation failure in medical patients undergoing invasive mechanical ventilation ranges from 3% to 19% (Epstein et al., 1997; Mador, 1998). This percentage seems to be much higher in neuromuscular diseases. One study published in 1997 reported that only half of patients were extubated within two weeks after intubation (Thomas et al., 1997). More recent studies indicate that extubation failure still occurs in more than 25% of these patients (Rabinstein and Mueller-Kronast, 2005; Seneviratne et al., 2008). Reintubaton is a significant event because these patients have significantly longer ICU and hospital stays (Rabinstein and Mueller-Kronast, 2005). Extubation failure is also associated with a higher incidence of ventilator-associated pneumonia (VAP) (Wu et al., 2009). Atelectasis is the most important risk factor for extubation failure in myasthenic crisis. Two retrospective studies found atelectasis in all patients requiring reintubation (Rabinstein and Mueller-Kronast, 2005; Seneviratne et al., 2008). Other factors identified include older age, pneumonia, acidosis, decreased VC, and need for noninvasive ventilatory support are predictors of reintubation (Rabinstein and Mueller-Kronast, 2005; Seneviratne et al., 2008; Wu et al., 2008).

Cough power is a strong predictor for extubation success in neuromusclar diseases. Bach and Saporito have reported that all patients with a cough PEF < 160 L/min had to be reintubated within 48 hours, the most likely reason being airway congestion because of the lack of adequate cough assistance (Bach and Saporito, 1996). In addition, patients who had passed SBT but presented cough PEF of 60 L/min or less were nearly 5 times more likely to fail extubation compared with those with cough PEF higher than 60 L/min (Salam et al., 2004). In myasthenics, our data indicate that extubation failure is most commonly associated with a weak cough and inadequate airway clearance, and Pemax is useful in predicting cough strength after extubation (Wu et al., 2009).

### 8.7 Tracheostomy

Tracheostomy is generally not needed in myasthenic crisis because the duration of intubation is often less than 2 weeks. Tracheostomy placement ranges from 14 to 40% (Thomas et al., 1997; Rabinstein and Mueller-Kronast, 2005). In our retrospective analysis of 41 episodes, tracheostomy was performed in four (9.8 %) patients after being ventilated for a median duration of 26 days (range: 20 to 30 days) (Wu et al., 2009). All these four patients were finally liberated from mechanical ventilation (Wu et al., 2009). One rare condition in myasthenic crisis that often requires tracheostomy is severe upper airway obstruction due to bilateral vocal cord paralysis. Approximately 11 such cases have been been reported in the literature and tracheotomy was required in the majority of these patients (Hanson et al., 1996).

## 9. Role of non-invasive positive pressure ventilation (NIPPV)

### 9.1 Advantages of NIPPV in neuromuscular diseases

The application of NIPPV can augment airflow and prevents airway collapse and maintaining gas exchange by offering positive airway pressure both in the inhalation and exhalation phases of respiration. It has been applied successfully in slowly progressive neuromuscular diseases, such as Duchenne muscular dystrophy or amyotrophic lateral sclerosis (Seneviratne et al., 2008). NIPPV should be started at low pressures initially and then inspiratory pressure is gradually increased while monitoring tolerance, symptoms, and gas exchange. NIPPV is also increasingly being used to prevent extubation failure in these patients. A recent prospective study suggests that application of NIPPV, combined with assisted coughing after extubation, averts the need for reintubation or tracheostomy in patients with neuromuscular diseases and shortening their stay in the ICU (Vianello et al., 2011). It should be included in the routine approach to these patients at high risk for postextubation respiratory failure.

### 9.2 Contraindications and disadvantages of NIPPV

Contraindications remain to the application of NIPPV in the acute setting, including respiratory arrest, severe inability to protect the airway, uncontrollable airway secretions despite use of noninvasive aids, life-threatening hypoxemia, severely impaired mental status or agitation, hemodynamic or electrocardiographic instability, and bowel obstruction (Hill et al., 2011). In patients with bulbar involvement, air blowing through a mask can lead to aspirated secretions and great care must be taken when using this modality (Wu et al., 2009). Current evidence suggests that NIPPV should be used judiciously, if at all, in patients with postextubation respiratory failure (Aqarwal et al., 2007).

### 9.3 Application of NIPPV in myasthenic crisis

The definition of myasthenic crisis was introduced before NIPPV was widely applied to patients with hypercapnic respiratory failure. One common dilemma is whether to do immediate intubation in a patient presenting with warning signs of imminent respiratory failure or to start with NIPPV support. There are studies that lend some credence to its use in selected patients with myasthenic crisis. In 2002, Rabinstein et al. first reported their experience of using NIPPV in these patients. In their case series, NIPPV was well tolerated and the length of hospital stay was significantly reduced compared to those who were intubated (mean 7 ± 5 days vs. 23 ± 16 days; $p = 0.03$). Most failures (75%) occurred within the first 24 hours of NIPPV use (Rabinstein et al., 2002). Several subsequent reports suggest that NIPPV may be useful in preventing intubation as well as reintubation in these patients (Rabinstein and Wijdicks, 2002; Rabinstein and Wijdicks, 2003; Seneviratne et al., 2008; Wu et al., 2009). In 60 episodes of crisis in 52 patients, Seneviratne et al. reported that NIPPV was the initial method of ventilatory support in 24 episodes, and intubation was avoided in 14 of these episodes (Seneviratne et al., 2008). Patients treated initially with NIPPV require ventilatory support for a median of 4 days versus 9 days in those patients initially intubated. A recent report also indicate that patients undergoing NIPPV spend one-third less time in the ICU and in the hospital, and the predictor of NIPPV failure was a $PaCO_2$ level exceeding 45 mm Hg on NIPPV initiation (Seneviratne et al., 2008). One retrospective cohort study found that NIPPV was never aborted because of excessive respiratory secretions in myasthenics, and there was no difference in pulmonary complications between those supported with NIPPV and those supported with endotracheal intubation mechanical ventilation (Seneviratne et al., 2008). In our study, independent predictors of NIPPV success were a serum bicarbonate < 30 mmol/L and an APACHE (Acute Physiological And Chronic Health Evaluation) II score < 6 (Wu et al., 2009). Our experience also suggests that intubation should be performed if the patient on NIPPV has continued or worsening shortness of breath, tachypnea, or hypercapniea.

### 9.4 NIPPV to prevent reintubation

Early application of NIPPV after extubation can reduce the risk of respiratory failure and lowered mortality in hypercapnic patients with chronic respiratory disorders (Ferrer et al., 2009). Use of NIPPV to avoid reintubation in myasthenic crisis is well established but relatively uncommon practice (Saeed and Patel, 2011). Some studies reported that NIPPV prevented reintubation in 70% of patients (Wu et al., 2009; Rabinstein and Wijdicks, 2002). Randomized controlled trials on the technique should be conducted before concluding the overall beneficial outcome.

## 10. Role of negative pressure ventilation

In recent years, the development of more portable and flexible devices has resulted in the renewed interest in the use of negative pressure ventilation to minimise the complications associated with positive pressure ventilation. Many of these devices can make the patients more comfortable with the ability to talk, eat and breathe freely around the mandatory negative pressure breaths. For example, the latest generation of biphasic cuirass ventilators are versatile and the duration and pressure can be altered in both the inspiratory and expiratory phases, which can promote the removal of secretions by external high-frequency oscillation as well as expiratory (cough) assistance (Linton, 2005; Koto et al., 2009). For myasthenic patients with relatively normal pulmonary compliance and airway resistance, it makes good sense to try cuirass ventilation to achieve earlier extubation. It should also reduce the incidence of VAP and laryngeal injury. Patients can then be moved to a step down or intermediate care facility, or even home, until muscle strength recovers.

## 11. Outcome and prognosis

### 11.1 Mortality

Patients in myasthenic crisis have an excellent outcome if respiratory support can be provided adequately and in time. The prognosis of myasthenic crisis has substantially improved. During the early 1960s, respiratory care of these patients was transitioned from negative external pressure ventilation to positive pressure ventilation in an ICU. The mortality rate during hospitalization has decreased from 42% in the early 1960s to 6% by the late 1970s, between 3% and 10% in the early 1980s, and less than 3% in the 1990s. The median age at death also increased (Cohen and Younger, 1981). The rate of mortality has continued to decline after 1990, presumably because of improvements in respiratory care and availability of treatment options including IVIG and plasma exchange (Alshekhlee et al., 2009). Based on the data in the US from 2000 through 2005, the overall in-hospital mortality rate in patients with MG was 2.2%, being higher in patients with crisis (4.47%) (Alshekhlee et al., 2009). Older age and respiratory failure were the predictors of death, with adjusted odds ratios of 9.28 and 3.58, respectively (Alshekhlee et al., 2009). In that cohort, significantly higher occurrence of cardiac complications, sepsis, and deep vein thrombosis was observed among patients with crisis; however, none of these complications were independent predictors of death (Alshekhlee et al., 2009).

### 11.2 Duration of mechanical ventilation and prognosis

Prior reports indicated a median duration of intubation of 13 days or ICU stay of 14 days (Murthy et al., 2005; Tether, 1955). A recent study noted a shorter median length of hospital stay of 6 days. However, this duration was 17 days for myasthenic patients who underwent endotracheal intubation (Alshekhlee et al., 2009). Duration of intubation is an important predictor of functional outcome after crisis. About 25% of patients are extubated on hospital day 7, 50% by hospital day 13, and 75% by hospital day 31. Eighteen percent of patients will require discharge to a rehabilitation center (Alshekhlee et al., 2009). In a retrospective study of 73 episodes of crisis, risk factors for prolonged intubation include patient age over 50 years, preintubation serum bicarbonate levels above 30 mg/dL, and highest VC of less than 25 mL/kg during the first week of intubation (Thomas et al., 1997). The risk of prolonged intubation (i.e., >2 weeks) was 0% in patients with none of these risk factors, 20% in those with one risk factor, 50% in those with two risk factors, and 90% in those with three risk factors (Thomas et al., 1997). In another study, 77% of patients intubated for more than 2 weeks had functional dependence at discharge compared with 36% of patients intubated for less than 2 weeks.

| | |
|---|---|
| 1. | Referred for intensive care. |
| 2. | Initial step is stabilization of the airway |
| 3. | Adequate oxygenation and ventilation. |
| 4. | Airway protection if bulbar dysfunction to prevent aspiration. |
| 5. | NIPPV if no contraindications. |
| 6. | Monitor vital signs and repeated measurements of muscle strength (VC, PImax, SNIP, PEmax, peak cough flow…). |
| 7. | 20/30/40 rule to guide intubation ( symptoms and signs more important). |
| 8. | Elective rather than emergency intubation. |
| 9. | Recommended initial ventilator settings: tidal volume 10 mL/kg, PS 5-15 cm $H_2O$ and PEEP 5-15 cm $H_2O$, peak airway pressure < 40 cm $H_2O$ |
| 10. | Aggressive chest physiotherapy and airway clearance. |
| 11. | Evaluation for weaning when muscular strength is objectively improved. |
| 12. | Identify readiness for extubation by spontaneous breathing trials (T-piece, PS, automatic tube compensation...). |
| 13. | Close monitoring and airway toilet after extubation. Tracheostomy is generally not needed. |

Table 2. Summary of respiratory care for myasthenic crisis

## 12. Conclusion

Myasthenic crisis is a rare but potentially life-threatening medical emergency and the diagnosis should be clinically suspected. The muscles involved and the degree of weakness vary from patient to patient, and respiratory care of these patients presents a challenge for the critical care practioners. Although no single factor determines the need for respiratory support, all patients with questionable respiratory status should be admitted to the ICU. Certain tests of respiratory muscle strength may help to identify impending respiratory failure and allow elective rather than emergent intubation. When treated aggressively adequately, patients generally have good outcomes in current practice. Successful management of patients not only involves the pharmacological aspect but a major part is mechanical ventilation. There is a clear need for formal randomized controlled trial of NIPPV in these patients as it seems to be a promising approach. Patient selection and close monitoring, however, remain important for successful application of NIPPV in myasthenic crisis. Because management of crisis includes treatment of the underlying MG, it is apparent that there is an urgent need for cooperation between specialist chest physicians, neurologists and respiratory therapists to optimize the care of this particular population of patients.

## 13. References

Aggarwal, AN.; Agarwal, R. & Gupta, D. (2009). Automatic tube compensation as an adjunct for weaning in patients with severe neuroparalytic snake envenomation requiring mechanical ventilation: a pilot randomized study. *Respiratory Care* Vol.54, No.12, pp. 1697-1702 ISSN 0020-1324

Ahmed, S.; Kirmani, JF., Janjua, N., Alkawi, A., Khatri, I., Yahia, AM., Souyah, N. & Qureshi, AI. (2005). An update on myasthenic crisis. *Current Treatment Options in Neurology* Vol.7, No.2, pp. 129-141, ISSN 1092-8480

Alshekhlee, A.; Miles, JD., Katirji, B., Preston, DC., & Kaminski, HJ. (2009). Incidence and mortality rates of myasthenia gravis and myasthenic crisis in US hospitals. *Neurology* Vol.72, No.18, pp. 1548-1554, ISSN 0028-3878

Argov, Z. (2009). Management of myasthenic conditions: nonimmune issues. *Current Opinion in Neurology* Vol.22, No.5, pp. 493-497, ISSN 1350-7540

Allen, SM.; Hunt, B. & Green, M. (1985). Fall in vital capacity with posture. *British Journal of Diseases of the Chest* Vol.79, No.3, pp. 267-271, ISSN 0007-0971

Alshekhlee, A.; Miles, JD., Katirji, B., Preston, DC. & Kaminski, HJ. (2009). Incidence and mortality rates of myasthenia gravis and myasthenic crisis in US hospitals. *Neurology* Vol.72, No.18, pp. 1548-1554, ISSN 0028-3878

Bach, JR. (1995). Amyotrophic lateral sclerosis: predictors for prolongation of life by noninvasive respiratory aids. *Archives of Physical Medicine and Rehabilitation* Vol.76, No.9, pp. 828–832, ISSN 0003-9993

Bach, JR. & Saporito, LR. (1996). Criteria for extubation and tracheostomy tube removal for patients with ventilatory failure: a different approach to weaning. Chest. Vol.110, No.6, pp. 1566-1571, ISSN 0012-3692

Bae, JS.; Go, SM., & Kim, BJ. (2006). Clinical predictors of steroid-induced exacerbation in myasthenia gravis. Journal of clinical neuroscience : official journal of the Neurosurgical, Vol.13, No.10, pp. 1006-1010, ISSN 0967-5868

Brooks-Brunn, JA. (1995). Postoperative atelectasis and pneumonia: Risk factors. *American Journal of Critical Care* Vol.4, No.5, pp. 340-349, ISSN 1062-3264

Baraka, A. (1992). Anaesthesia and myasthenia gravis. *Canadian Iournal of Anaesthesia* Vol.39, pp. 476-486, ISSN 0832-610X

Berrouschot, J.; Bauman, I., Kalischewski, P., Sterker, M., & Schneider, D. (1997). Therapy of myasthenic crisis. *Critical Care Medicine* Vol.25, No.7, pp. 1228–1235 ISSN 0090-3493

Borel, CO.; Teitelbaum, JS. & Hanley, DF. (1993). Ventilatory drive and carbon dioxide response in ventilatory failure due to myasthenia gravis and Guillain–Barre syndrome. *Critical Care Medicine* Vol.21, No.11, pp. 1717–1726, ISSN 0090-3493

Bedlack, RS. & Sanders, DB. (2002). On the concept of myasthenic crisis. *Journal of Clinical Neuromuscular Disease* Vol.4, No.1, pp. 40-42 ISSN 1522-0443

Chaudhuri, A. & Behan, PO. (2009). Myasthenic crisis. *QJM* Vol.102, No.2, pp. 97-107 ISSN 1460-2725

Chatwin, M. & Simonds, AK. (2009). The addition of mechanical insufflation/ exsufflation shortens airway-clearance sessions in neuromuscular patients with chest infection. *Respiratory Care* Vol.54, No.11, pp. 1473-1479 ISSN 0020-1324

Chatwin, M.; Ross, E., Hart, N., Nickol, AH., Polkey, MI. & Simonds, AK. (2003). Cough augmentation with mechanical insufflation/exsufflation in patients with neuromuscular weakness. *European Respiratory Journal* Vol.21 No.3, pp. 502–508 ISSN 0903-1936

Cohen, MS. & Younger, D. (1981). Aspects of the natural history of myasthenia gravis: crisis and death. *Annals of the New York Academy of Sciences* Vol.377, pp. 670-677, ISSN 0077-8923

Crescimanno, G.; Marrone, O. & Vianello, A. (2011). Efficacy and comfort of volume-guaranteed pressure support in patients with chronic ventilatory failure of neuromuscular origin. *Respirology* Vol.16, No.4, pp. 672-679 ISSN 1323-7799

Dushay, KM., Zibrak, JD. & Jensen, WA. (1990). Myasthenia gravis presenting as isolated respiratory failure. *Chest* Vol.97, No.1, pp. 232-234, ISSN 0012-3692

Elsais, A.; Johansen, B. & Kerty, E. (2010). Airway limitation and exercise intolerance in well-regulated myasthenia gravis patients. *Acta Neurologica Scandinavica Supplementum* Vol.190, pp. 12-17, ISSN 0065-1427

Ely, EW.; Baker, AM., Dunagan, DP., Burke, HL., Smith, AC., Kelly, PT., Johnson, MM., Browder, RW., Bowton, DL. & Haponik, EF. (1996). Effect on the duration of mechanical ventilation of identifying patients capable of breathing spontaneously. *New England Journal of Medicine* Vol.335, No.25, pp. 1864–1869, ISSN 0028-4793

Ely, EW.; Bennett, PA., Bowton, DL., Murphy, SM., Florance, AM. & Haponik, EF. (1999). Large scale implementation of a respiratory therapist-driven protocol for ventilator weaning. *American Journal of Respiratory and Critical Care Medicine* Vol.159, No.2, pp. 439–446, ISSN 1073-449X

Epstein, SK.; Ciubotaru, RL. & Wong, JB. (1997). Effect of failed extubation on the outcome of mechanical ventilation. *Chest* Vol.112, No.1, pp. 186-192 , ISSN 0012-3692

Esteban, A.; Alía, I., Gordo, F., Fernández, R., Solsona, JF., Vallverdú , I., Macías, S., Allegue, JM., Blanco, J., Carriedo, D., León, M., de la Cal, MA., Taboada, F., Gonzalez de Velasco, J., Palazón, E., Carrizosa, F., Tomás, R., Suarez, J. & Goldwasser, RS. (1997). Extubation outcome after spontaneous breathing trials with T-tube or pressure support ventilation. The Spanish Lung Failure Collaborative Group.

*American Journal of Respiratory and Ccritical Care Medicine* Vol.156, No.2 pt 1, pp. 459–465, ISSN 1073-449X

Fabry, B.; Guttmann, J., Eberhard, L. & Wolff, G. (1994). Automatic compensation of endotracheal tube resistance in spontaneously breathing patients. *Technology and Health Care* Vol.1, pp. 281-291, ISSN 0928-7379

Ferrer, M.; Sellarés, J., Valencia, M., Carrillo, A., Gonzalez, G., Badia, JR., Nicolas, JM. & Torres A. (2009). Noninvasive ventilation after extubation in hypercapnic patients with chronic respiratory disorders: randomised controlled trial. *Lancet* Vol.374, No,9695, pp. 1082-1088, ISSN 0140-6736

Friedman, S. & Goffin, FB. (1966). Abductor vocal weakness in myasthenia gravis: report of a case. *Laryngoscope* Vol. 76, No.9, pp. 1520-1523, ISSN 0023-852X

García Río F, Prados C, Díez Tejedor E, Díaz Lobato S, Alvarez-Sala R, Villamor J, Pino JM. (1994). Breathing pattern and central ventilatory drive in mild and moderate generalised myasthenia gravis. *Thorax* Vol.49, No.7, pp. 703-706, ISSN 0040-6376

Garcia-Pachon, E.; Casan, P. & Sanchis, J. (1996). Myasthenia gravis and upper airway dysfunction. *Chest* Vol.110, No.4, pp. 1127-1128, ISSN 0012-3692

Gracey, DR.; Divertie, MB., Howard, FM Jr. (1983). Mechanical ventilation for respiratory failure in myasthenia gravis. Two-year experience with 22 patients. *Mayo Clinic Proceedings* Vol.58, No.9, pp. 597–602, ISSN 0025-6196

Hanson; JA.; Lueck, CJ., Thomas, DJ. (1996). Myasthenia gravis presenting with stridor. *Thorax* Vol.51, No.1. pp. 108-109, ISSN 0040-6376

Hardy, KA. & Anderson, BD. (1996). Noninvasive clearance of airway secretions. *Respiratory Care Clinics of North America* Vol.2, No.2, pp. 323-345, ISSN 1078-5337

Hart, N.; Polkey, MI., Sharshar, T., Falaize, L., Fauroux, B., Raphaël, JC. & Lofaso, F. (2003). Limitations of sniff nasal pressure in patients with severe neuromuscular weakness. *Journal of Neurology, Neurosurgery and Psychiatry* Vol.74, No.12, pp. 1685-1687, ISSN 0022-3050

Hill, NS.; Brennan, J., Garpestad, E.& Nava, S. (2007). Noninvasive ventilation in acute respiratory failure. *Critical Care Medicine* Vol.35, No.10, pp. 2402-2407, ISSN 0090-3493

Hudspeth, MP.; Holden, KR. & Crawford, TO. (2006). The "slurp" test: bedside evaluation of bulbar muscle fatigue. *Pediatrics* Vol.118, No.2, pp: e530-533, ISSN 1098-4275

Jaretzki, A 3rd,; Barohn, RJ., Ernstoff, RM., Kaminski, HJ., Keesey, JC., Penn, AS. & Sanders, DB. (2000). Myasthenia gravis: recommendations for clinical research standards. Task Force of the Medical Scientific Advisory Board of the Myasthenia Gravis Foundation of America. *Neurology* Vol.55, No.1, pp. 16-23, ISSN 0028-3878

Juel, VC. (2004). Myasthenia gravis: management of myasthenic crisis and perioperative care. *Seminars in Neurology* Vol.24, No.1, pp. 75-81, ISSN 0271-8235

Kato, K.; Sato, N., Takeda, S., Yamamoto, T., Munakata, R., Tsurumi, M., Suzuki, D., Yagi, K., Tanaka, K. & Mizuno, K. (2009). Marked improvement of extensive atelectasis by unilateral application of the RTX respirator in elderly patients. *Internal Medicine* Vol.48, No.16, pp. 1419-1423, ISSN 0918-2918

Keesey, JC. (2004). Clinical evaluation and management of myasthenia gravis. *Muscle and Nerve* Vol.29, No.4, pp. 484-505, ISSN 0148-639X

Kelly, BJ. & Luce, JM. (1991). The diagnosis and management of neuromuscular diseases causing respiratory failure. *Chest* Vol.99, No.6, pp. 1485–1494, ISSN 0012-3692

Kirmani, JF.; Yahia, AM. & Qureshi, AI. (2004). Myasthenic crisis. *Current Treatment Options in Neurology* Vol.6, No.1, pp. 3-15, ISSN 1092-8480

Lacomis, D. (2005) Myasthenic crisis. *Neurocritical Care* Vol.3, No.3, pp. 189-194, ISSN 1541-6933

Lewis, FR. (1980). Management of atelectasis and pneumonia. *The Surgical Clinics of North America* Vol. 60, No.6, pp. 1391–1401, ISSN 0039-6109

Liggett, SB.; Daughaday, CC., Senior, RM. (1988). Ipratropium in patients with COPD receiving cholinesterase inhibitors. *Chest* Vol.94, No.1, pp. 210-212, ISSN 0012-3692

Linton, DM. (2005). Cuirass ventilation: a review and update. *Critical Care and resuscitation* Vol.7, No.1, pp. 22–28, ISSN 1441-2772

Mador, MJ. (1998). Weaning from mechanical ventilation: what have we learned and what do we still need to know? *Chest* Vol.114, No.3, pp.672-674, ISSN 0012-3692

Mayer, SA. (1997). Intensive care of the myasthenic patient. *Neurology* Vol.48, No.Suppl5, pp. S70-S75, ISSN 0028-3878

Martínez-Llorens, J.; Ausín, P., Roig, A., Balañá, A., Admetlló, M., Muñoz, L. & Gea, J. (2011). Nasal inspiratory pressure: an alternative for the assessment of inspiratory muscle strength? *Archivos de Bronconeumología* Vol.47, No.4, pp. 169-175, ISSN 0300-2896

Mier-Jedrzejowicz, AK.; Brophy, C. & Green, M. (1988). Respiratory muscle function in myasthenia gravis. *American Review of Respiratory Disease* Vol.138, No.4, pp. 867-873, ISSN 0003-0805

Mier, A.; Laroche, C. & Green, M. (1990). Unsuspected myasthenia gravis presenting as respiratory failure. *Thorax* Vol.45, No.5, pp.422-423, ISSN 0040-6376

Murthy, JM.; Meena, AK., Chowdary, GV.& Naryanan JT. (2005). Myasthenic crisis: clinical features, complications and mortality. *Neurology India* Vol.53, No.1, pp. 37–40, ISSN 0028-3886

Nocturnal oxygen therapy trial group. (1980). Continuous or nocturnal oxygen therapy in hypoxemic chronic obstructive lung disease: a clinical trial *Annals of Internal Medicine* Vol.93, No.3, pp. 391-398, ISSN 0013-4819

Namen, AM.; Ely, EW., Tatter, SB., Case, LD., Lucia, MA, Smith A, Landry S, Wilson JA, Glazier SS, Branch CL, Kelly DL, Bowton DL & Haponik, EF. (2001). Predictors of successful extubation in neurosurgical patients. *American Journal of Respiratory and Critical Care Medicine* Vol.163, pp. 658-664, ISSN 1073-449X

No authors. (1991). AARC (American Association for Respiratory Care) clinical practice guideline: Incentive spirometry. *Respiratory Care* Vol.36, No.12, pp. 1402–1405, ISSN 0020-1324

O'Riordan, JI.; Miller, DH., Mottershead, JP., Hirsch, NP. & Howard RS. (1998). The management and outcome of patients with myasthenia gravis treated acutely in a neurological intensive care unit. *European Journal of Neurology* Vol.5, No.2, pp. 137-142, ISSN 1351-5101

Pascuzzi, RM., Coslett, HB. & Johns, TR. (1984). Long-term corticosteroid treatment of myasthenia gravis: report of 116 patients. *Annals of Neurology* Vol.15, No.3, pp. 291-298, ISSN 0364-5134

Perez, T. (2006). Neuromuscular disorders - assessment of the respiratory muscles. *Revue Neurologique* Vol.162, No.4, pp. 437-444, ISSN 0035-3787

Phillips LH. The epidemiology of myasthenia gravis. (2004). *Seminars in Neurology* Vol.24, No.1, pp. 17-20. ISSN 0271-8235

Plauche, WC. (1991). Myasthenia gravis in mothers and their newborns. *Clinical Obstetrics and Gynecology* Vol.34, No.1, pp. 82-99, ISSN 0009-9201

Prigent H, Orlikowski D, Letilly N, Falaize L, Annane D, Sharshar T, Lofaso F. (2011). Vital capacity versus maximal inspiratory pressure in patients with Guillain-Barré syndrome and myasthenia gravis. *Neurocrit Care* Jul 12. [Epub ahead of print], ISSN 1541-6933

Phillips, LH 2nd. & Torner JC. (1996). Epidemiologic evidence for a changing natural history of myasthenia gravis. *Neurology* Vol.47, No.5, pp. 1233–1238, ISSN 0028-3878

Polkey, MI.; Lyall, RA., Green, M., Nigel Leigh, P. & Moxham J. (1998). Expiratory muscle function in amyotrophic lateral sclerosis. *American Journal of Respiratory and Critical Care Medicine* Vol.158, No.3, pp. 734–741, ISSN 1073-449X

Prigent, H.; Lejaille, M., Falaize, L., Louis, A., Ruquet, M., Fauroux, B., Raphael, JC. & Lofaso F. (2004). Assessing inspiratory muscle strength by sniff nasal inspiratory pressure. *Neurocrit Care* Vol.1, No.4, pp. 475-478 ISSN 1541-6933

Putman, MT. & Wise, RA. (1996). Myasthenia gravis and upper airway obstruction. *Chest* Vol.109, No.2, pp. 400-404, ISSN 0012-3692

Rabinstein A, Wijdicks EF. (2002). BiPAP in acute respiratory failure due to myasthenic crisis may prevent intubation. *Neurology* Vol.59, No.10, pp. 1647-1649, ISSN 0028-3878

Rabinstein, AA. & Wijdicks, EF. (2003). Weaning from the ventilator using BiPAP in myasthenia gravis. *Muscle and Nerve* Vol.27, No.2, pp. 252-253, ISSN 0148-639X

Rabinstein, AA. & Mueller-Kronast, N. (2005) Risk of extubation failure in patients with myasthenic crisis. *Neurocrit Care* Vol.3, No3, pp. 213-215, ISSN 1541-6933

Rabinstein, AA. & Wijdicks, EF. (2003). Warning signs of imminent respiratory failure in neurological patients. *Seminars in Neurology* Vol.23, No.1, pp. 97-104, ISSN 0271-8235

Rieder, P., Louis, M., Jolliet, P. & Chevrolet, JC. (1995). The repeated measurement of vital capacity is a poor predictor of the need for mechanical ventilation in myasthenia gravis. *Intensive Care Medicine* Vol.21, No.8, pp. 663-668, ISSN 0342-4642

Saeed, T. & Patel, S. (2011). Use of non invasive ventilation to avoid re-intubation in myasthenia gravis; a case report and review of literature. *Journal of the Pakistan Medical Association* Vol.61, No.3, pp. 293-295, ISSN 0030-9982

Salam, A.; Tilluckdharry, L., Amoateng-Adjepong, Y. & Manthous CA. (2004). Neurologic status, cough, secretions and extubation outcomes. *Intensive Care Medicine* Vol.30, No.7, pp. 1334-1339, ISSN 0342-4642

Selsby, D. & Jones, JG. (1990) Some physiological and clinical aspects of chest physiotherapy. *British Journal of Anaesthesia* Vol.64, No.5, pp. 621–631, ISSN 0007-0912

Seneviratne, J.; Mandrekar, J., Wijdicks, EF. & Rabinstein, AA. (2008). Predictors of extubation failure in myasthenic crisis. *Archives of Neurology* Vol.65, No.7, pp. 929-933, ISSN 0003-9942

Seneviratne, J.; Mandrekar, J., Wijdicks, EF.& Rabinstein, AA. (2008). Noninvasive ventilation in myasthenic crisis. *Archives of Neurology* Vol.65, No.1, pp. 54-58, ISSN 0003-9942

Soliman, MG.; Higgins, SE., El-Kabir, DR., Davidson, AC., Williams, AJ. & Howard, RS. (2005). Non-invasive assessment of respiratory muscle strength in patients with previous poliomyelitis. *Respiratory Medicine* Vol.99, No.10, pp. 1217–1222, ISSN 0954-6111

Steier, J.; Kaul, S., Seymour, J., Jolley, C., Rafferty, G., Man, W., Luo, YM., Roughton, M., Polkey, MI. & Moxham, J. (2007). The value of multiple tests of respiratory muscle strength. *Thorax* Vol.62, No.11, pp. 975–980, ISSN 0040-6376

Suárez, AA.; Pessolano, FA., Monteiro, SG., Ferreyra, G., Capria, ME., Mesa, L., Dubrovsky, A. & De Vito, EL. (2002). Peak flow and peak cough flow in the evaluation of expiratory muscle weakness and bulbar impairment in patients with neuromuscular disease. *American Journal of Physical Medicine and Rehabilitation* Vol.81, No.7, pp. 506-511, ISSN 0894-9115

Szathmáry, I.; Magyar, P. & Szobor, A. (1981). Myasthenia gravis: protective effect of ipratropium bromide (Atrovent) on airways obstruction caused by edrophonium chloride (Tensilon). *European Neurology* Vol.20, No.1, pp. 56-61, ISSN 0014-3022

Thomas, CE.; Mayer, SA., Gungor, Y., Swarup, R., Webster, EA., Chang, I., Brannagan, TH., Fink, ME. & Rowland LP. (1997). Myasthenic crisis: clinical features, mortality, complications, and risk factors for prolonged intubation. *Neurology* Vol.48, No.5, pp. 1253-1260, ISSN 0028-3878

Toussaint, M.; De Win, H., Steens, M. & Soudon P. (2003). Effect of intrapulmonary percussive ventilation on mucus clearance in duchenne muscular dystrophy patients: a preliminary report. *Respiratory Care* Vol.48, No.10, pp. 940-947, ISSN 0020-1324

Varelas,PN.; Chua, HC., Natterman, J., Barmadia, L., Zimmerman, P., Yahia, A., Ulatowski, J., Bhardwaj, A., Williams, MA. & Hanley, DF. (2002). Ventilatory care in myasthenia gravis crisis: assessing the baseline adverse event rate. *Critical Care Medicine Vol.*30, pp. 2663-2668, ISSN 0090-3943

Vianello, A.; Donà, A., Salvador, V. & Ori C. (2010). Extubation of patients with neuromuscular weakness: a routine step or a challenging procedure? *Chest* Vol.138, No.4, pp. 1026-1027, ISSN 0012-3692

Vianello, A.; Arcaro, G., Braccioni, F., Gallan, F., Marchi, MR., Chizio, S., Zampieri, D., Pegoraro, E. & Salvador V. (2011). Prevention of extubation failure in high-risk patients with neuromuscular disease. *Journal of Critical Care Vol.26, pp. 517–524,* ISSN 1557-8615

Windisch, W.; Hennings, E., Sorichter, S., Hamm, H. & Criée, CP. (2004). Peak or plateau maximal inspiratory mouth pressure: which is best? *The European Respiratory Journal* Vol.23, pp. 708–713, ISSN 0903-1936

Wendell, LC. & Levine, JM. (2011) Myasthenic Crisis. *The Neurohospitalist* Vol.1, pp. 16-22, ISSN 1941-8744

Wilson, SR.; Quantz, MA., Strong, MJ. & Ahmad, D. (2005). Increasing peak expiratory flow time in amyotrophic lateral sclerosis. *Chest* Vol.127, No.1, pp.156-160, 0012-3692

Wu, JY.; Kuo, PH., Fan, PC., Wu, HD., Shih, FY. & Yang, PC. (2009). The role of non-invasive ventilation and factors predicting extubation outcome in myasthenic crisis. *Neurocrit Care* Vol.10, No.1, pp. 35-42, ISSN 1541-6933

# Part 3

## Surgical Considerations

6

# Unilaterally Extended Thoracoscopic Thymectomy: The Right Side or the Left Side Approach

Victor Tomulescu
*Fundeni Clinical Institute, Center of General Surgery and Liver Transplant "Dan Setlacec"*
*Romania*

## 1. Introduction

Myasthenia gravis (MG) is a heterogeneous disorder with a protean, clinical, pathologic, and immunobiological picture(Beekman, Kuks, and Oosterhuis 1997, 244:112-118) Myasthenia gravis (MG) is the best studied and understood autoimmune disease. The autoimmune origin of the disease was suggested for the first time by Simpson (Simpson 1982, 226:1045-1050), but Almon and colleagues(Almon and Appel 1976, 274:235-243) were the first to demonstrate circulating antibodies to acetylcholine receptor (AchR) sites of the neuromuscular junction. Elevated antibody levels are found in approximately 90% of patients and are roughly correlated with the clinical severity of the disease(Beekman, Kuks, and Oosterhuis 1997, 244:112-118). As Lennon (Lennon, Lindstrom, and Seybold 1976, 274:283-299) showed, the thymus is evidently implicated in the production not only of these end-plate antibodies but also to striated muscle antibodies through some aberration in its normal function.

In most cases, the target of the autoimmune attack is the nicotinic acetylcholine receptor (AChR) located in the postsynaptic muscle endplate membrane. AChR antibodies produce deficient neuromuscular transmission by three different mechanisms:

- they bind to the AChR and alter function;
- they promote endocytosis and accelerate the degradation rate of AchR
- antibodies activate complement leading to destruction of the postsynaptic surface(Hughes, Moro De Casillas, and Kaminski 2004, 24:21-30).

Other neuromuscular junction antigens, distinct from AChR, also play a role in autoimmune attack of patients with MG. Up to 20% of patients with generalized MG are seronegative for AChR antibodies with 30% of these patients having autoantibodies directed against a distinct endplate membrane intrinsic protein, muscle-specific receptor tyrosine kinase (MuSK) (Evoli et al. 2003, 126:2304-2311). Some MuSK antibodies compromise AChR channel function, but specific pathogenic mechanisms have not been defined. One would predict that MuSK antibodies compromise neuromuscular transmission by affecting AChR clustering at the neuromuscular jonction. Patients who have late onset non-tumoral MG may also have tintin (an intracellular muscle protein) and ryanodine receptor antibodies, the presence of these antibodies being associated with a worse prognosis (Romi, Gilhus, and Aarli 2006, 183:24-25).

The thymus plays a key role in tolerance induction to self-antigens and in responsiveness of lymphocytes to foreign antigens. Several findings indicate that the thymus is involved in MG pathogenesis:

- Pathological changes, like lymphoid follicular hyperplasia or thymomas, are frequent in patients with MG.
- MG thymic tissue contains abnormally elevated amounts of mature T cells, most of them AChR-reactive T cells(Sommer et al. 1990, 28:312-319;Sommer, Tackenberg, and Hohlfeld 2008, 91:169-212).
- myasthenic thymic tissue fragments transplanted to severe combined immunodeficiency mice produce human antibodies, which bind to the AChR(Schonbeck et al. 1992, 90:245-250).

Most myasthenic thymuses contain B cells capable of producing AchR antibodies, particularly those hyperplastic thymuses with germinal centers(Leite et al. 2007, 171:893-905). Normal and myasthenic human thymuses express gene transcripts and epitopes of all AchR As subunits(Navaneetham et al. 2001, 24:203-210).

The availability of AChR in thymus may play a role in pathogenesis of MG. It is considered that the AChR expressed on thymic myoid cells is the original auto-sensitizing antigen, and the thymic changes in MG are primary events in the autoimmune pathogenesis of the disease(Leite, Jones, Strobel, Marx, Gold, Niks, Verschuuren, Berrih-Aknin, Scaravilli, Canelhas, Morgan, Vincent, and Willcox 2007, 171:893-905). It is possible that the myoid cells to be altered by viral illness involving the thymus and the proximity to antigen presenting cells and helper T-cells to facilitate the abnormal immunologic response(Drachman 1994, 330:1797-1810).

Patients with MG have frequently other immune-mediated diseases like rheumatoid arthritis, lupus, Graves' disease, tyroiditis and a family history of autoimmune disorders. That imposed the study of the genetic factor implication in MG. HLA types like HLA-B8, DRw3, Dqw2 have been associated with AChR antibody positive MG and haplotypes DR14 and DQ5 with MuSK antibody positive MG(Carlsson et al. 1990, 31:285-290;Niks et al. 2006, 66:1772-1774).

Since the first case reported by Schumacher and Roth in 1913 (Keesey 2004, 24:5-16), the role of thymectomy in MG treatment has been well established. The main study demonstrating the benefit of thymectomy in MG was that of Buckingham and associates(Buckingham et al. 1976, 184:453-458), who compared the clinical course of patients after thymectomy with a computer-matched cohort receiving medical therapy. The best assessment of potential benefits of thymectomy in modern era comes from a review of 21 controlled but non-randomized studies(Gronseth and Barohn 2000, 55:7-15) showing that patients undergoing thymectomy were twice as likely to achieve medication-free remissions.

## 2. Indication (thymectomy in the multimodal treatment of MG)

The major issues for a surgeon who has an interest in thymectomy are related to patient selection and surgical technique. Regarding patient selection, decision should be taken in cooperation with the neurologist that supervised the treatment. Coordinated and strong multidisciplinary collaboration among neurologists, surgeons and anaesthesiologists is mandatory in making appropriate decisions regarding patient selection, therapeutic options and the timing of surgery.

There is a current consensus that a patient with generalized non-tumoral MG who is between puberty and 60 years of age should undergo surgery, but the optimal approach is still under debate(Toyka KV and Gold R 2007, 158:309-321). Surgery for patients older than 60 years is controversial. In patients with ocular myasthenia the benefit is uncertain (Bulkley et al. 1997, 226:324-334;Guillermo et al. 2004, 109:217-221)

Nowadays surgical procedures for thymectomy in non-tumoral MG comprise transternal, transthoracic, transcervical, subxifoidian or thoracoscopic thymectomy. The primary goal of every technique, of every surgeon doing thymectomy is "to remove as much thymus and ectopic thymus as possible"(Rubin 2006, 82:1007-1008). An optimal approach should combine least invasiveness and maximal radicality.

This is related with Jaretski's (Jaretzki, Steinglass, and Sonett 2004, 24:49-62;Jaretzki, III and Wolff 1988, 96:711-716) now classic point of view in relation to thymus anatomy: that the main body of the gland, incapsulated consisting in a right and a left lobe that join at their central portion just caudal to the left innominate vein, is accompanied with small extracapsular foci of thymic tissue distributed widely in mediastinal and cervical adipose tissue. This is the reason why the surgical technique consists in rigorous emptying of the anterior mediastinum from diaphragm to the cervical area, between the phrenic nerves, of all thymus and fatty tisuue. Advantages of thoracoscopic thymectomy besides minimizing the trauma and undoubted cosmetic advantages consist in the exceptional intraoperative overview (the new high definition cameras make these images even more accurate) that make the procedure safer, and diminishing the risk of injury of fine structures not related with the procedure.

The diagnosis of myasthenia gravis is based on the patient's history, physical examination, positive response to anticholinesterase agents and electrophysiology studies. Preoperative diagnostic tests should include spirometry and a CT scan. The immunologic profile with AchR antibodies assay and anti-MuSK antibody should be performed on all patients. Thymectomy should be performed when MG is in a stable condition; there is no indication for "emergency operation". Al the patients should be well prepared for the intervention. In our experience patients were considered suitable for a surgical procedure only when evidence showed good treatment tolerance and a decrease of the quantitative myasthenia gravis score (Myastenia Gravis Foundation of America (MGFA) recommendations for clinical research standards (Jaretzki, III et al. 2000, 70:327-334)) to at least 10 points.

Unilaterally extended thoracoscopic thymectomy is performed with the patient under general anesthesia with double-lumen tube placement and lying in a 15-30° off-centre position (fig1).

Choice of the side is matter of training, mentoring, safe complete removal of the thymus and peri-thymic fatty tissue from diaphragm to cervical area being the main goal. A versatile thoracic surgeon should be able to approach the thymus by a variety of methods and if a left side approach is not possible due to previous thoracotomy for example, a right side approach should be performed with the same dexterity, safety and preciseness.

## 3. Left side approach or right side approach

Three or four trocars are inserted into the left hemithorax. The operator stays on the left side of the patient in a caudal position to the cameraman, but these positions are not fixed and any improvement in better ergonomics or superior visualization should be taking into account. The monitor is on the right side of the patient. The first trocar (10–12 mm) is placed through the fifth or sixth intercostal space, between the middle and posterior axillar lines.

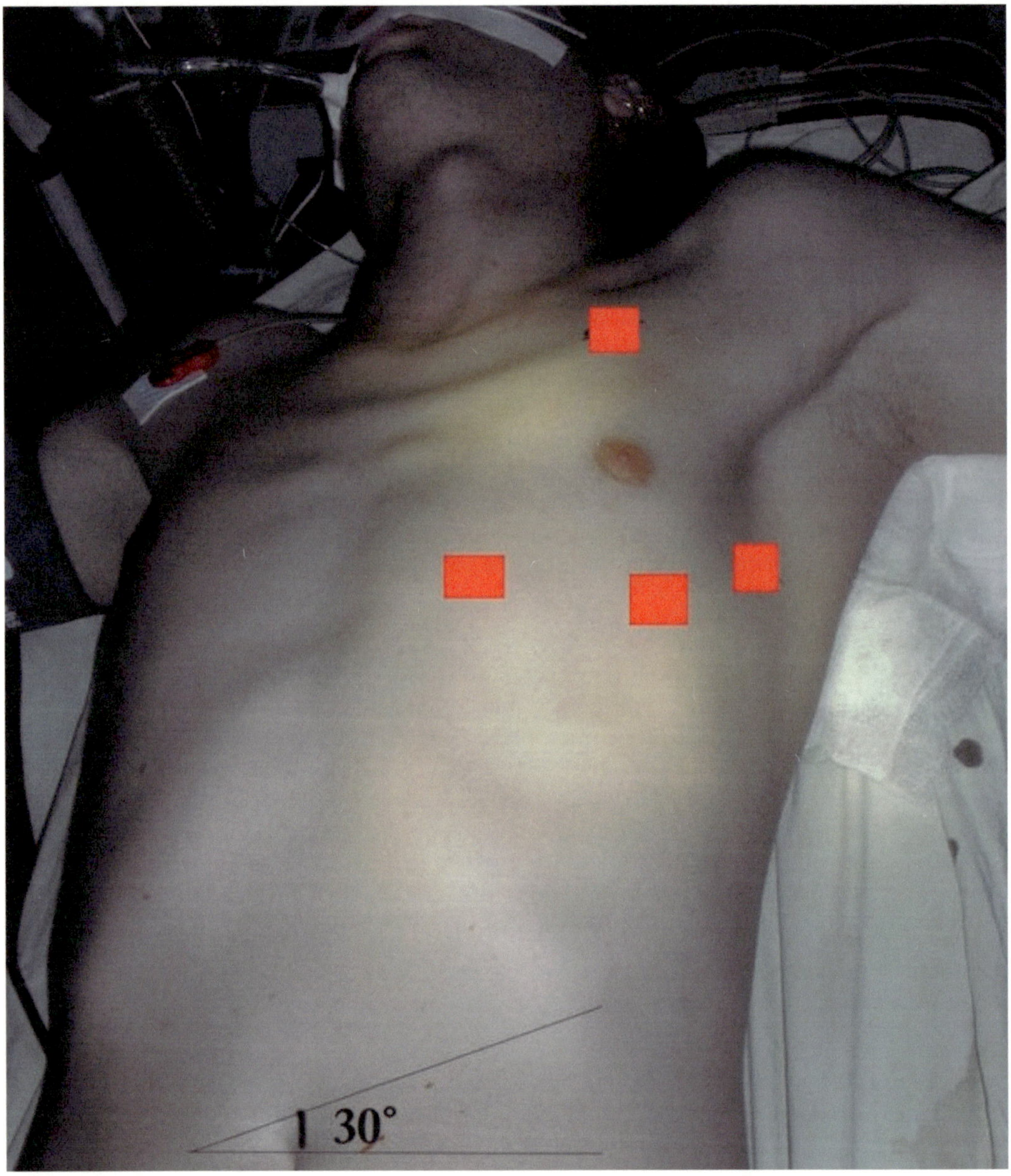


Fig. 1. Patient and trocar positioning

Pleural cavity exploration is facilitated by the selective right bronchus intubation and by $CO_2$ insufflations at a maximum of 10 mmHg pressure (fig2).

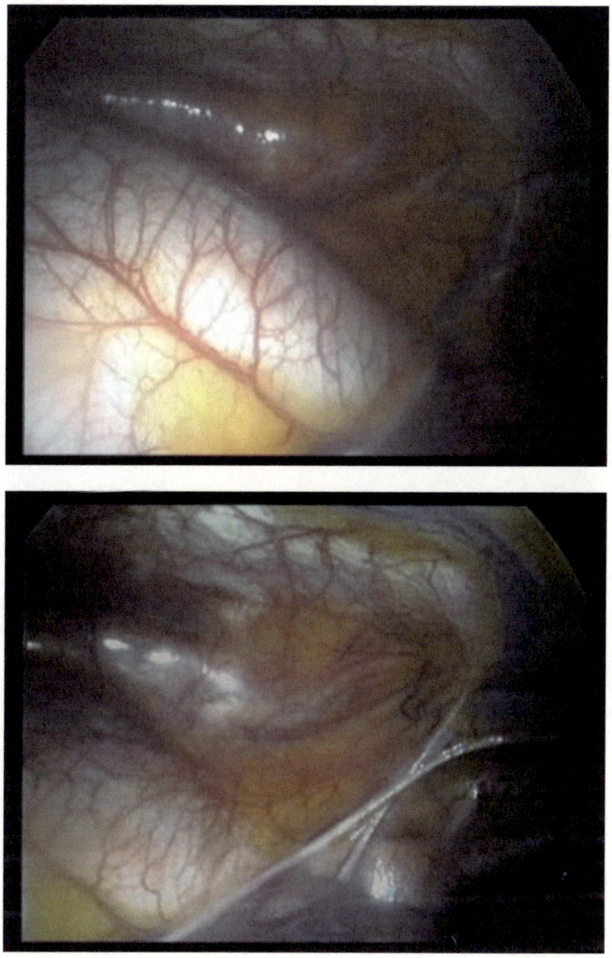

Fig. 2. $CO_2$ insufflations at a maximum of 10 mmHg pressure enlarge the anterior mediastinum space

The second and third trocars (10–12 and 5–7 mm or 10-12mm, respectively) are placed through the third inter-costal space on the anterior axilary line and through the fourth or fifth inter-costal spaces on the mid-clavicle line. For females the incision should be done keeping in mind the important cosmetic problem of the peri -mammary scars.

After a careful pleural cavity exploration we spot the anterior mediastinum. The capnotorax helps us also in the dissection. In order to have this support we need to start all the operations with incision of the mediastinal pleura along the two important landmarks of thymectomy: the phrenic nerve and the internal thoracic artery (fig3), allowing the gas dissection to help us.

The incision of the mediastinal pleura and the dissection of the thymus begin anterior to the left phrenic nerve and continue into the entire thymus compartment. The use of the ultrascision scalpel (Harmonic Scalpel Ultrascision; Ethicon Endo-Surgery) facilitates the dissection, decreases the time of the intervention, and avoids the risks of the electrocoagulation in this area. The cranial limit of the dissection, at the level of the mediastinal pleura, is the internal thoracic artery. The operation continues with dissection of the inferior left thymic horn and pericardial fatty tissue (fig 4).

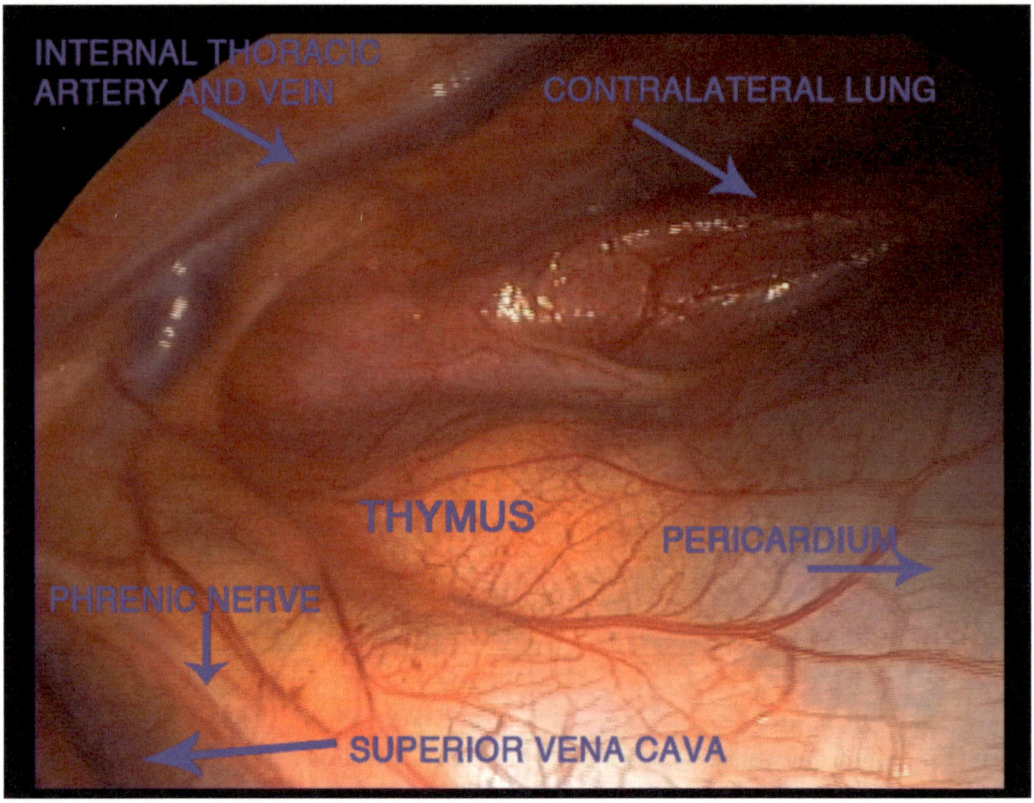


Fig. 3. Landmarks of the anterior mediastinum in thymectomy (right side approach)

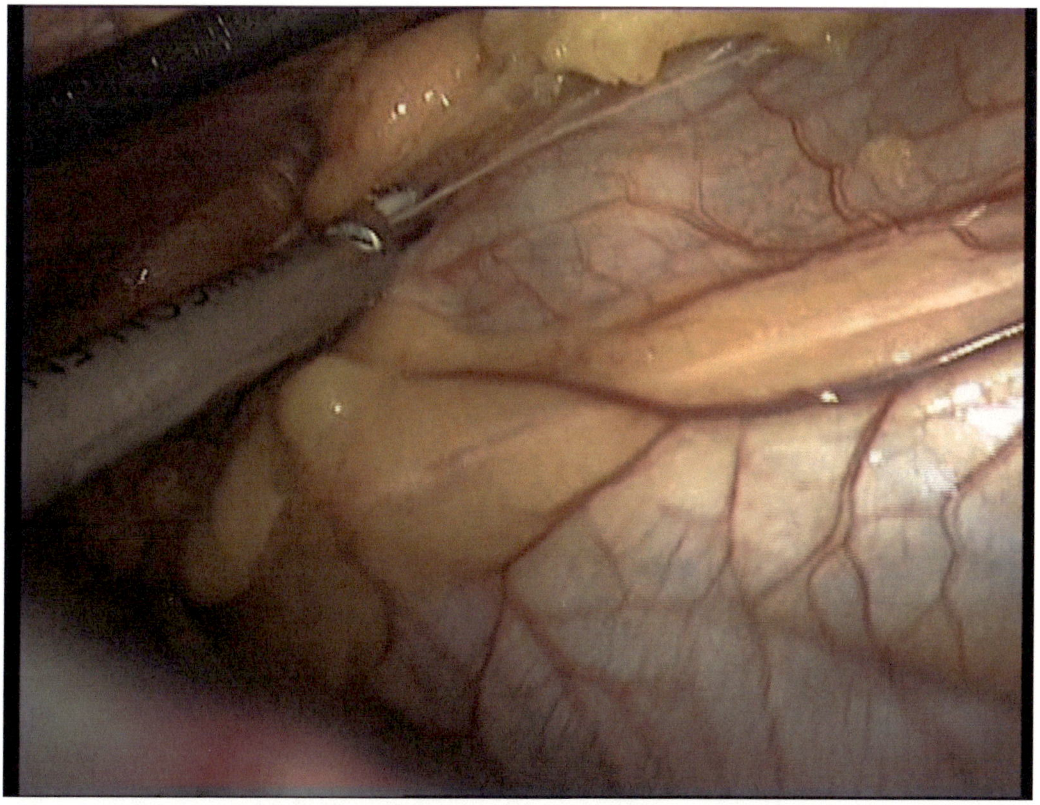

Fig. 4. Dissection of the left inferior thymus horn - beginning of the intervention

The dissection of the thymic tissue together with pericardial fat goes cephalad on the pericardial plane (fig5) overtaking the median line, to the right of the thymus gland. The contra-laterally mediastinal pleura is opened and the inferior right thymic horn and pericardial fatty tissue is dissected in the same manner (fig6). We continue to dissect anterior, retrosternal, the mediastinal pleura being open on the right side till the right mammary pedicle. The posterior dissection continues similar, the pericardium, the aortic arch, the left brachiocephalic vein, and the superior vena cava are visualized and cleaned of all fat tissue or thymus. The most difficult area to dissect is in the aortopulmonary window (fig 7) and the aortocaval groove (fig 8). At the superior pole, the dissection is performed in the anterior carotidal plane to the internal thoracic artery level. The left superior horn or some time both upper horns may occasionally pass behind, instead of in front of the brahiocephalic vein (fig 9). This anatomical variety is more difficult to be solved by thoracoscopic approach. We have to be aware of the vagus nerve ant left recurrent laryngeal nerve that goes close and dissect carefully inferior and posterior to the brahiocephalic vein and then superior, to free the cervical parts of the upper horns. Afterwards traction of the upper horns caudally permits the dissection of them behind the brahiocephalic vein, in order to visualize an eventual posterior thymus vein.

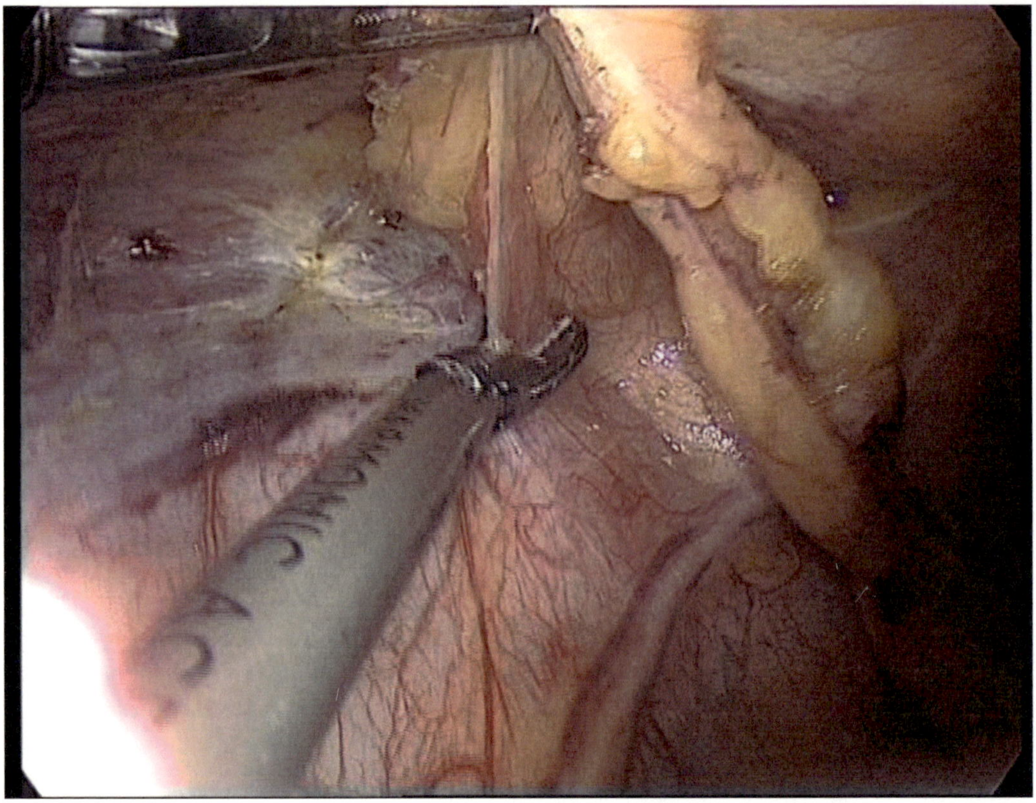

Fig. 5. Dissection in the pre-pericardial plane

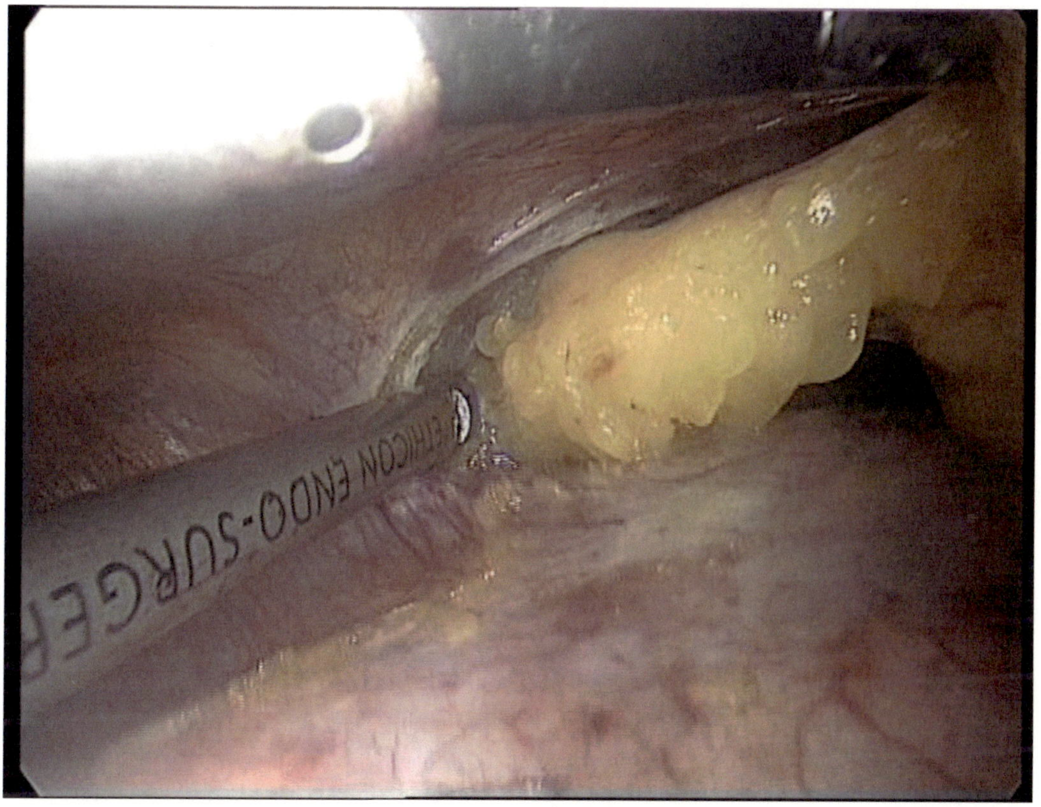


Fig. 6. Dissection of the contra-laterally inferior horn (left side approach)

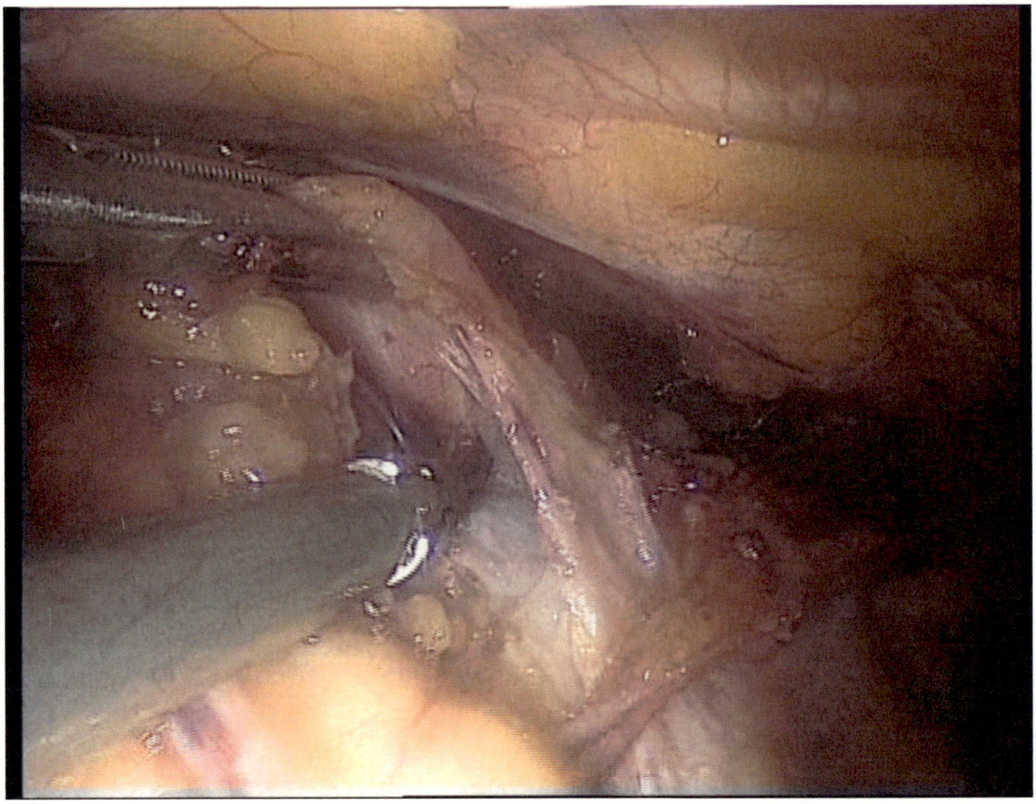

Fig. 7. Dissection of the aortopulmonary window

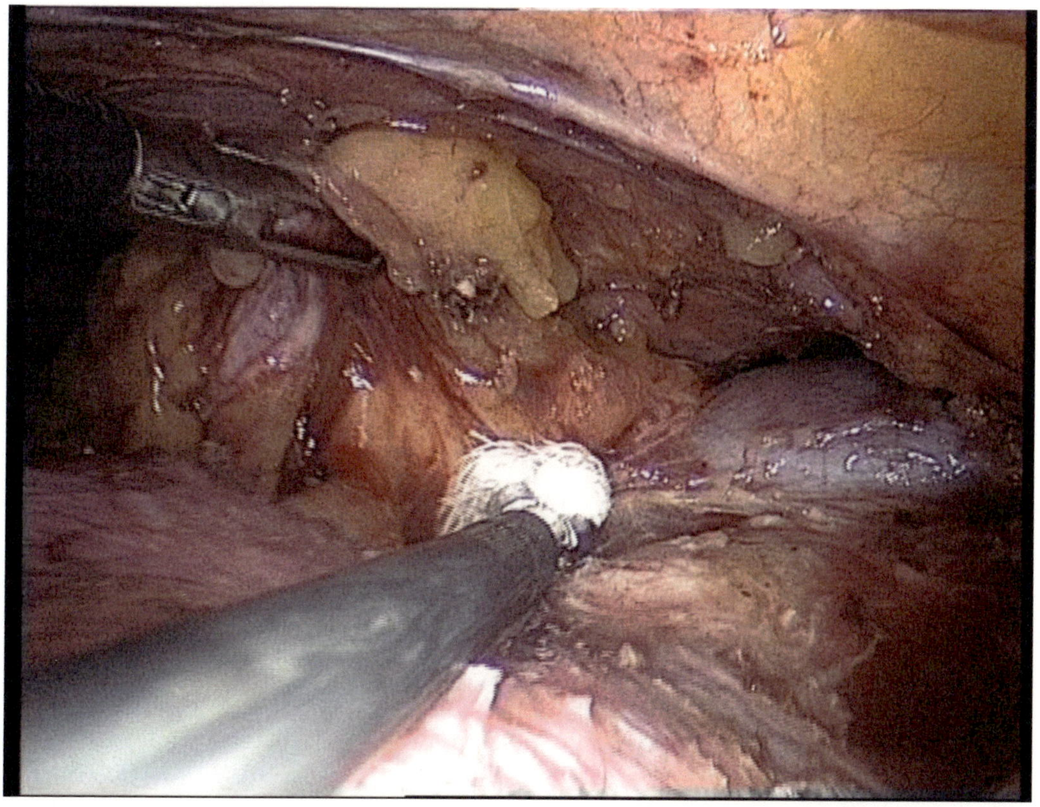

Fig. 8. Dissection of the aorto-caval groove

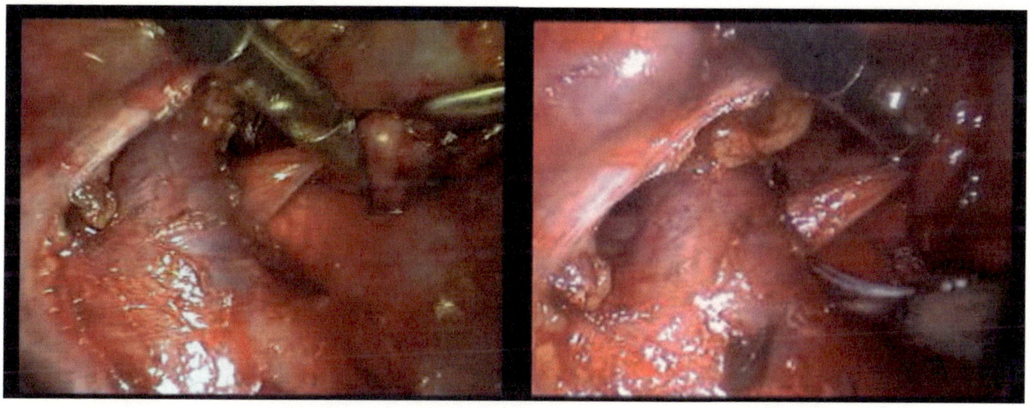

Fig. 9. Posterior upper right thymus horn dissection (right side approach)

The thymectomy ends with the identification of the superior part of the gland, the thyroid-thymic ligament section, and freeing of the superior horns from the surrounding tissue. After dissecting the surrounding fascia and cutting the vessels that goes caudally from cervix, upper horns can be mobilized caudally by applying gentle traction (fig 10). Cervical skin transillumination is the indication that the cervical limit of the dissection has been reached. During the operation, we can visualize the superior, lateral, or medial arterial thymic pedicles. They are clipped and cut or ultrasonically coagulated (fig 11). Dissection of the thymic veins is very important. The veins are very short and enter directly into the left brachiocephalic vein. Tearing out such a pedicle may cause a hemorrhage, which is very difficult to correct thoracoscopically. Visualization of the right phrenic nerve is necessary to complete the dissection of thymus and fatty tissue (fig 12).

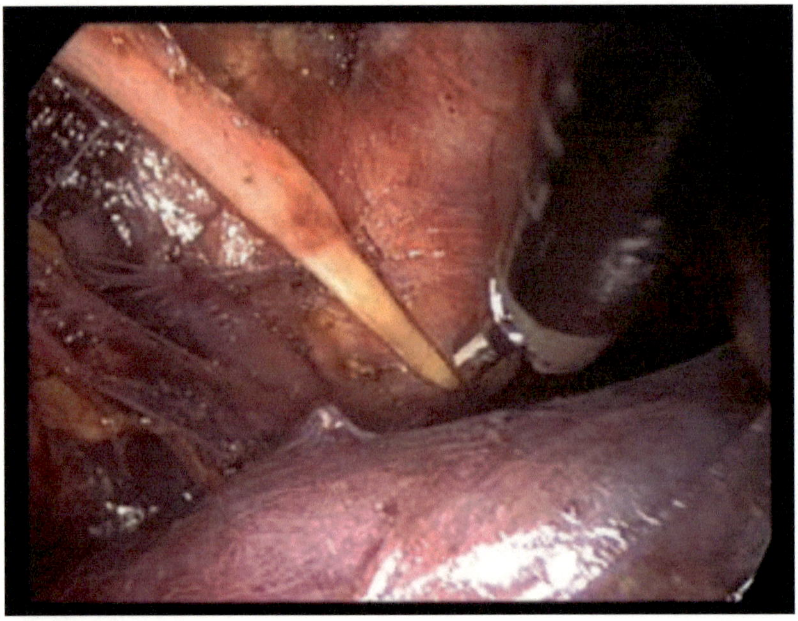

Fig. 10. Dissection of the upper left horn

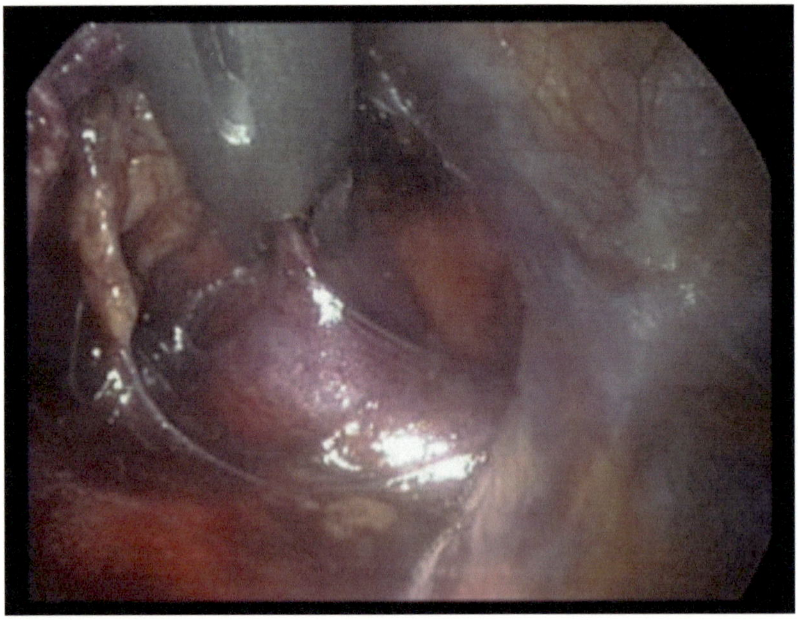

Fig. 11. Clipping the thymus vein

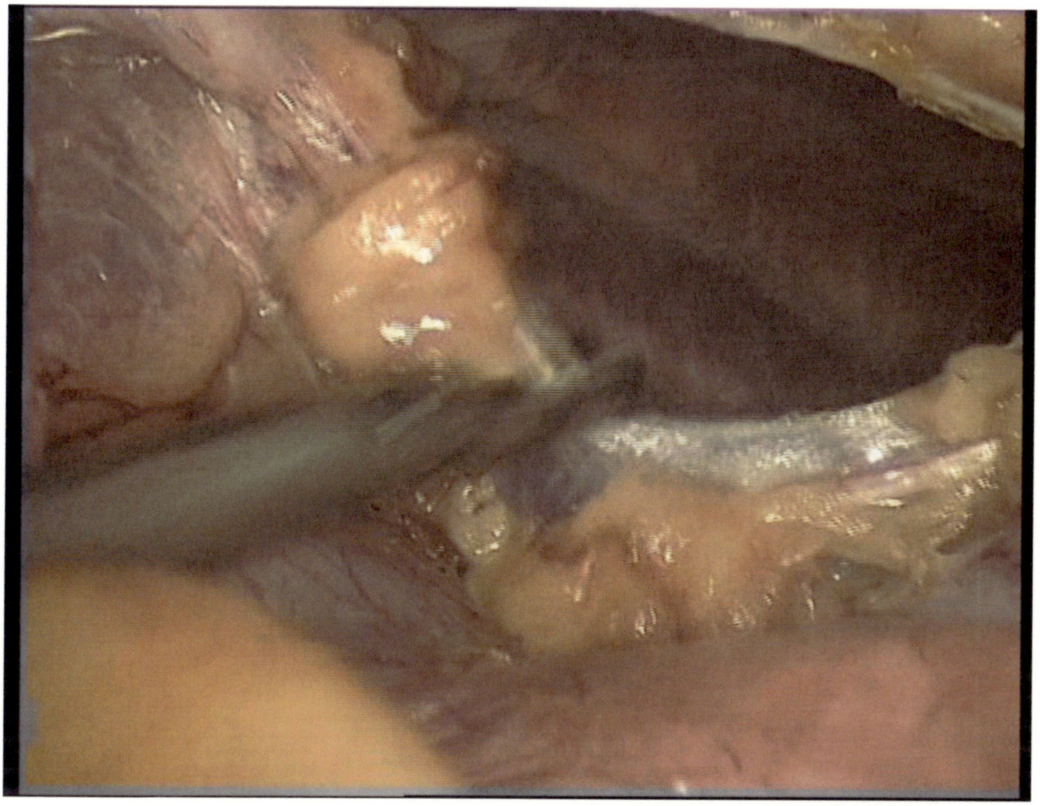

Fig 12. Visualization of the right phrenic nerve (left side approach)

We sometimes used a needle-scope camera that was inserted through the Veress needle in the contra lateral thorax to control the complete dissection (fig 13).

Thymus extraction is quite easily done by enlarging the hole of one of the trocar ports and bagging the piece before extracting it (fig 14). We prefer to introduce the bag at the beginning of the intervention, this way any small piece of thymus or fatty tissue could be bagged during dissection.

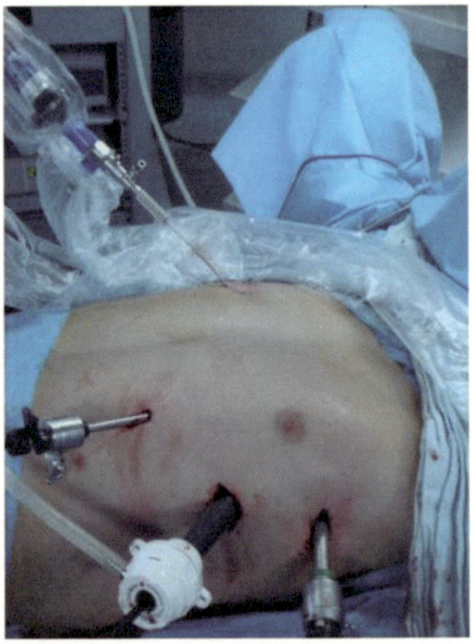

Fig. 13. Control of the complete dissection with a needle-scope camera that was inserted through the Veress needle in the contra lateral thorax

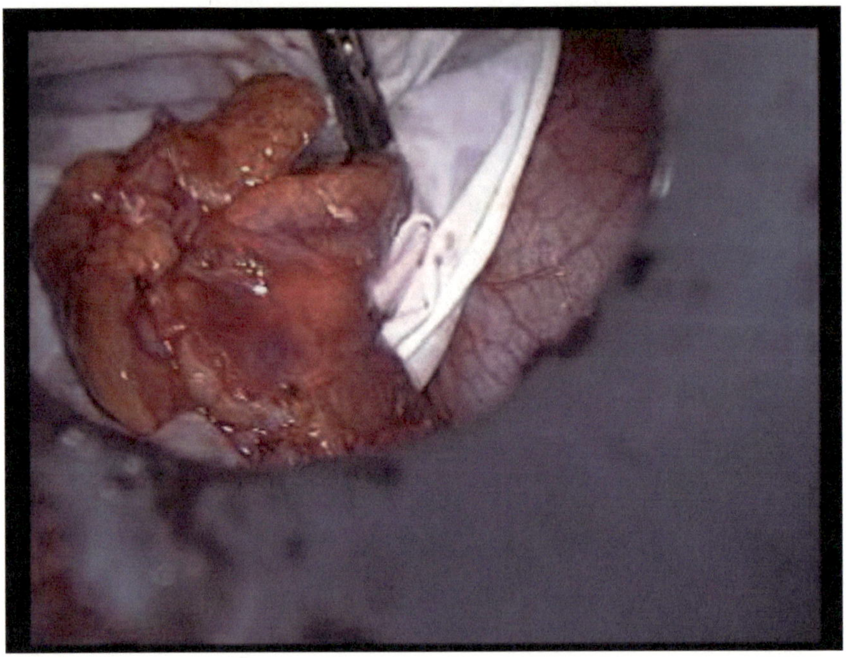

Fig. 14. Extractic the specimen in self-made bag

The operation ends with the thymic cavity inspection, which can detect possible remnant tissue (fig 15). Finally, we wash the cavity with warm saline. At the end of the operation one or two drains can be placed in the pleural cavity through the inferior trocar ports.

Thoracoscopic thymectomy through the right side is performed in the same manner, the most difficult part of this approach being the aortopulmonary window(Ruckert et al. 2000, 18:735-736) and left inferior horn.

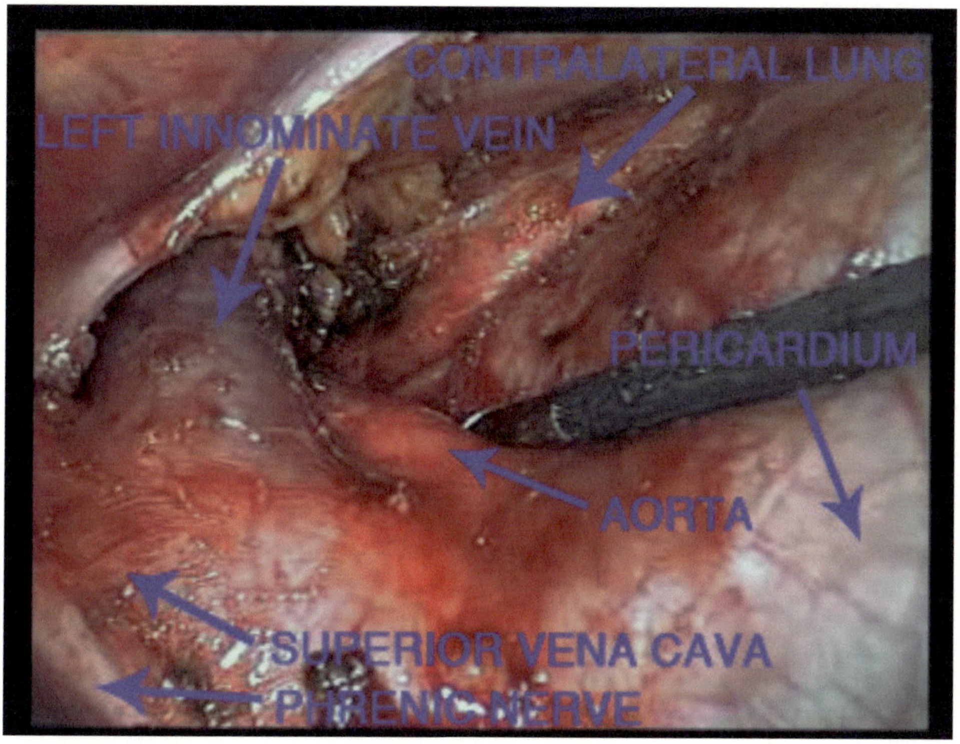


Fig 15. Landmarks of the anterior mediastinum at the end of thymectomy (right side approach)

Yim and colleagues(Yim 1997, 64:584-585) favor the right thoracoscopic approach because:

1. identification of the vena cava is a landmark for easier dissection of innominate vein,
2. the confluence of the innominate veins is easier to dissect by using a right approach,
3. ergonomically, it is easier for right-hand surgeons to dissect the thymus from inferior horns to upper horns with a right approach.

To this we would add that the right approach allows a better view in the cervical area. Irrespective of the patient's anatomic characteristics, every effort is made to perform a full removal of the thymic tissue by clearing the innominate vein and anterior pericardium from all mediastinal fat. We believe a left-side approach facilitates the procedure because most of the mediastinal fat is located on the left side of the anterior mediastinum. The use of a 30° endoscope (Karl Storz-Endoscopy) provides significant help. Although we share the opinion of Mineo and colleagues(Mineo, Pompeo, and Ambrogi 1997, 114:516-517) that thymectomy can be performed by either a left-side or a right-side approach, we believe the left-side approach has some advantages. In our experience, the dissection maneuvers are safer when performed on the left side because the right phrenic nerve is situated outside the surgical field, thus reducing the risk of an incidental lesion. It is also easier to perform a dissection of the right side of the thymus by a left approach than a dissection of the left side of the thymus by right approach, especially for the aortopulmonary window.

## 4. Personal results

Since April 1999, a thoracoscopic approach has been used in all patients admitted in the Department of General Surgery and Liver Transplantation of Fundeni Clinical Institute with either nonthymomatous myasthenia gravis or stage I and IIa Masaoka thymomas. There have been 300 patients with nontumoral myasthenia gravis (NTMG) that have suffered an extended thoracoscopic thymectomy in our center between April 1998 and April 2011.

We considered that favourable outcomes requires highly coordinated teamwork involving a strong collaboration between neurologists, surgeons, and anesthesiologists in making appropriate decisions on selection of patients, therapeutic options, and timing of surgery. All of the patients received specific treatment for at least 3 months before surgery in the Department of Neurology of our institute. Patients were considered suitable for a surgical procedure only when evidence showed good treatment tolerance and a stable quantitative myasthenia gravis (QMG) score of at least 10 points. We did not operate patients with pure ocular myasthenia gravis because we considered that the indication for thymectomy in ocular myasthenia gravis remained controversial. We did not operate patients with age over 60 years.

Treatment, morbidity, mortality, and postinterventional status at follow-up were also assessed according to the MGFA Recommendations for Clinical Research Standards, QMG scores being the most valuable tool in quantitative evaluation of clinical improvement or remission analysis. CSR was used as the end point for the evaluation of the efficacy and prognostic factors. Patients were considered to be in complete stable remission status if they exhibited no symptoms of MG for at least one year and had received no therapy for MG during that time.

A left thoracoscopic approach was used for 29% of the patients and a right thoracoscopic approach for 71% of the patients. Decision to use the right-side or left-side approach was considered in relation with the CT aspect of each patient's thymus. Extensive dissection in the region of the thyroid and lateral neck, through a separate collar incision, was not routinely performed. The low probability of finding aberrant thymic remnants in these locations did not justify this approach as a standard procedure. Minicervicotomies were performed on 7 patients, due to cervical extensions of the thymus. There were no conversions to open thymectomy. The mean operative time was of 80+/- 45 min. There was zero mortality and morbidity was observed in 14 patients (4.66%): 10 patients previously reported(Tomulescu et al. 2006, 82:1003-1007) (severe postoperative myasthenia crisis in 1 patient who needed mechanical ventilation for 5 days, 2 with contralateral pneumothorax after drain removal, 3 with hemothorax that required emergent reintervention, and 6 with prolonged pleural drainage) and 2 patients with postoperative pneumonia.

The mean length of hospitalization was 2.1 days (range: 2-6 days).

Evaluating the post-interventional status according to the MGFA recommendations for Clinical Research Standards complete stabile remission (CSR) have been obtained in 62% (186 patients), pharmacologic remission (PR) in 8% (24 patients), minimal manifestation (MM) in 15% (45 patients), non changed (N) in 10% (30 patients), worse (W) in 1% (3 patients) and exacerbation (E) - patients who have fulfilled the criteria of CSR, PR, or MM but subsequently developed clinical findings greater than permitted by these criteria - in 4% (12 patients).

## 5. Conclusions

Unilaterally extended thoracoscopic thymectomy is a technically demanding procedure that requires expertise in extended thymectomy and in advanced minimally invasive techniques. The right side, the left side or even bilateral approach should be chosen in relation with the method the surgeon is more comfortable and from which best results (morbidity, mortality, completeness of thymectomy) should be expected.

The maximal thymectomy should remain the benchmark against which other thymectomy techniques are measured (whether or not it is the surgical technique of choice) (Jaretzki, III, Barohn, Ernstoff, Kaminski, Keesey, Penn, and Sanders 2000, 70:327-334;Jaretzki, III and Wolff 1988, 96:711-716; Sonett and Jaretzki, III 2008, 1132:315-328) but we consider that with no mortality, low morbidity, comparable CSR and PR, better cosmetic and pulmonary function-sparing effect, superior compliance from the patients and neurologists with a higher rate acceptance of surgical treatment, this minimally invasive approach could become the best first solution in the multimodal treatment of myasthenia gravis.

## 6. References


Almon RR, and Appel SH. 1976. Serum acetylcholine-receptor antibodies in myasthenia gravis. *Ann. N. Y. Acad. Sci.* 274: 235-243.

Beekman R, Kuks JB, and Oosterhuis HJ. 1997. Myasthenia gravis: diagnosis and follow-up of 100 consecutive patients. *J. Neurol.* 244 (2): 112-118.

Buckingham JM, Howard FM, Jr., Bernatz PE, Payne WS, Harrison EG, Jr., O'Brien PC, and Weiland LH. 1976. The value of thymectomy in myasthenia gravis: a computer-assisted matched study. *Ann. Surg.* 184 (4): 453-458.

Bulkley GB, Bass KN, Stephenson GR, Diener-West M, George S, Reilly PA, Baker RR, and Drachman DB. 1997. Extended cervicomediastinal thymectomy in the integrated management of myasthenia gravis. *Ann. Surg.* 226 (3): 324-334.

Carlsson B, Wallin J, Pirskanen R, Matell G, and Smith CI. 1990. Different HLA DR-DQ associations in subgroups of idiopathic myasthenia gravis. *Immunogenetics* 31 (5-6): 285-290.

Drachman DB. 1994. Myasthenia gravis. *N. Engl. J. Med.* 330 (25): 1797-1810.

Evoli A, Tonali PA, Padua L, Monaco ML, Scuderi F, Batocchi AP, Marino M, and Bartoccioni E. 2003. Clinical correlates with anti-MuSK antibodies in generalized seronegative myasthenia gravis. *Brain* 126 (Pt 10): 2304-2311.

Gronseth GS, and Barohn RJ. 2000. Practice parameter: thymectomy for autoimmune myasthenia gravis (an evidence-based review): report of the Quality Standards Subcommittee of the American Academy of Neurology. *Neurology* 55 (1): 7-15.

Guillermo GR, Tellez-Zenteno JF, Weder-Cisneros N, Mimenza A, Estanol B, Remes-Troche JM, and Cantu-Brito C. 2004. Response of thymectomy: clinical and pathological characteristics among seronegative and seropositive myasthenia gravis patients. *Acta Neurol. Scand.* 109 (3): 217-221.

Hughes BW, Moro De Casillas ML, and Kaminski HJ. 2004. Pathophysiology of myasthenia gravis. *Semin. Neurol.* 24 (1): 21-30.

Jaretzki A, III, Barohn RJ, Ernstoff RM, Kaminski HJ, Keesey JC, Penn AS, and Sanders DB. 2000. Myasthenia gravis: recommendations for clinical research standards. Task Force of the Medical Scientific Advisory Board of the Myasthenia Gravis Foundation of America. *Ann. Thorac. Surg.* 70 (1): 327-334.

Jaretzki A, Steinglass KM, and Sonett JR. 2004. Thymectomy in the management of myasthenia gravis. *Semin. Neurol.* 24 (1): 49-62.

Jaretzki A, III, and Wolff M. 1988. "Maximal" thymectomy for myasthenia gravis. Surgical anatomy and operative technique. *J. Thorac. Cardiovasc. Surg.* 96 (5): 711-716.

Keesey JC. 2004. A history of treatments for myasthenia gravis. *Semin. Neurol.* 24 (1): 5-16.

Leite MI, Jones M, Strobel P, Marx A, Gold R, Niks E, Verschuuren JJ, Berrih-Aknin S, Scaravilli F, Canelhas A, Morgan BP, Vincent A, and Willcox N. 2007. Myasthenia gravis thymus: complement vulnerability of epithelial and myoid cells, complement attack on them, and correlations with autoantibody status. *Am. J. Pathol.* 171 (3): 893-905.

Lennon VA, Lindstrom JM, and Seybold ME. 1976. Experimental autoimmune myasthenia gravis: cellular and humoral immune responses. *Ann. N. Y. Acad. Sci.* 274: 283-299.

Mineo TC, Pompeo E, and Ambrogi V. 1997. Video-assisted thoracoscopic thymectomy: from the right or from the left? *J. Thorac. Cardiovasc. Surg.* 114 (3): 516-517.

Navaneetham D, Penn AS, Howard JF, Jr., and Conti-Fine BM. 2001. Human thymuses express incomplete sets of muscle acetylcholine receptor subunit transcripts that seldom include the delta subunit. *Muscle Nerve* 24 (2): 203-210.

Niks EH, Kuks JB, Roep BO, Haasnoot GW, Verduijn W, Ballieux BE, De Baets MH, Vincent A, and Verschuuren JJ. 2006. Strong association of MuSK antibody-positive myasthenia gravis and HLA-DR14-DQ5. *Neurology* 66 (11): 1772-1774.

Romi F, Gilhus NE, and Aarli JA. 2006. Myasthenia gravis: disease severity and prognosis. *Acta Neurol. Scand. Suppl* 183: 24-25.

Rubin JW. 2006. Invited commentary. *Ann. Thorac. Surg.* 82 (3): 1007-1008.

Ruckert JC, Czyzewski D, Pest S, and Muller JM. 2000. Radicality of thoracoscopic thymectomy--an anatomical study. *Eur. J. Cardiothorac. Surg.* 18 (6): 735-736.

Schonbeck S, Padberg F, Hohlfeld R, and Wekerle H. 1992. Transplantation of thymic autoimmune microenvironment to severe combined immunodeficiency mice. A new model of myasthenia gravis. *J. Clin. Invest* 90 (1): 245-250.

Simpson JA. 1982. Myasthenia gravis. *Practitioner* 226 (1368): 1045-1050.

Sommer N, Tackenberg B, and Hohlfeld R. 2008. The immunopathogenesis of myasthenia gravis. *Handb. Clin. Neurol.* 91: 169-212.

Sommer N, Willcox N, Harcourt GC, and Newsom-Davis J. 1990. Myasthenic thymus and thymoma are selectively enriched in acetylcholine receptor-reactive T cells. *Ann. Neurol.* 28 (3): 312-319.

Sonett JR, and Jaretzki A, III. 2008. Thymectomy for nonthymomatous myasthenia gravis: a critical analysis. *Ann. N. Y. Acad. Sci.* 1132: 315-328.

Tomulescu V, Ion V, Kosa A, Sgarbura O, and Popescu I. 2006. Thoracoscopic thymectomy mid-term results. *Ann. Thorac. Surg.* 82 (3): 1003-1007.

Toyka KV, and Gold R. 2007. Treatment of myasthenia gravis. *Schweiz Arch Neurol Psychiatr* 158: 309-321.

Yim AP. 1997. Thoracoscopic thymectomy: which side to approach? *Ann. Thorac. Surg.* 64 (2): 584-585.

# 7

# Robotic Thymectomy

Victor Tomulescu
*Fundeni Clinical Institute, Center of General Surgery and Liver Transplant "Dan Setlacec"*
*Romania*

## 1. Introduction

After the great success of minimally invasive approach in abdominal surgery, thoracoscopic surgery has gained a broad acceptance for diagnostic and therapeutic procedures due to the fact that permits good exposure of the pleural cavity, enables extensive dissection and combines the advantages of minimal invasive surgery with little tissue trauma, short recovery, less pain and improved cosmetic results.

Although thoracoscopic surgery brings clear benefits to the patients, surgeons face distinct disadvantages: working through fixed entry points limits maneuverability of the instruments inside the body cavity, looking at a two-dimensional screen. Surgeons are handicapped by the loss of the visual depth perception, the need for a human assistant to hold and move the camera makes surgeons lose the independent ability of controlling the operation field (Vasilescu C and Popescu I 2008, 103:9-11).

Telemanipulator robots have been developed in response to limitations placed on the surgeon by endoscopic surgery: reduced visual quality and control, reduced dexterity related to the instrumentation, ergonomics.

Of the two advanced surgical robotic systems that are used for thoracic and abdominal surgery only "da Vinci" remains since the 2003 acquisition of Computer Motion by Intuitive Surgical and the corporate decision to stop production of the Zeus system.

The Da Vinci system consists of three primary components: the surgeon's viewing and control console (fig 1),a movable cart with three or four articulated robot arms (fig2) and the camera tower(the vision cart) (fig3).

The console is located outside the sterile field. The surgeon is seated in front of the console and manipulates handles that are similar to "joysticks" while viewing a high-resolution, truly three-dimensional image of the surgical field through binoculars (fig 4). Manipulation of the handles transmits electronic signals to the computer, which can control and modify the movement of instrument tips by downscaling the movements, by eliminating physiologic tremor, and by adjusting grip strength applied to the tools. The masters are aligned with instrument tips, making the movement of the instruments natural and intuitive. The surgeon can also monitor the status of the instruments and arms without removing the head from the console through the various messages that are displayed on the display. In fact the sensation is that messages appear in the operation field. An infrared sensor disable the robotic arms as soon as the surgeon removes his/her head from the console. The computer generates electrical impulses that are transmitted by a 10 meter long cable and command the three or four articulated robot arms. The surgeon is using the masters to manipulate the instruments and the camera but also the foot pedals to clutch, camera clutch, electrocautery or ultrasonic shears control.

Disposable laparoscopic articulated instruments are attached to the distal part of two arms or three in the four arm robot and introduced inside or the thorax through trocars mounted on the arms. One of the arms carries an endoscope with dual optical channels, one channel for each of the surgeon's eyes. The camera and instrument arms are attached to the column of the surgical cart. The arms are draped with specific sterile drapes before intervention. Each instrument arm and the camera arm is draped separately and instrument arm adapters are attached (fig5).

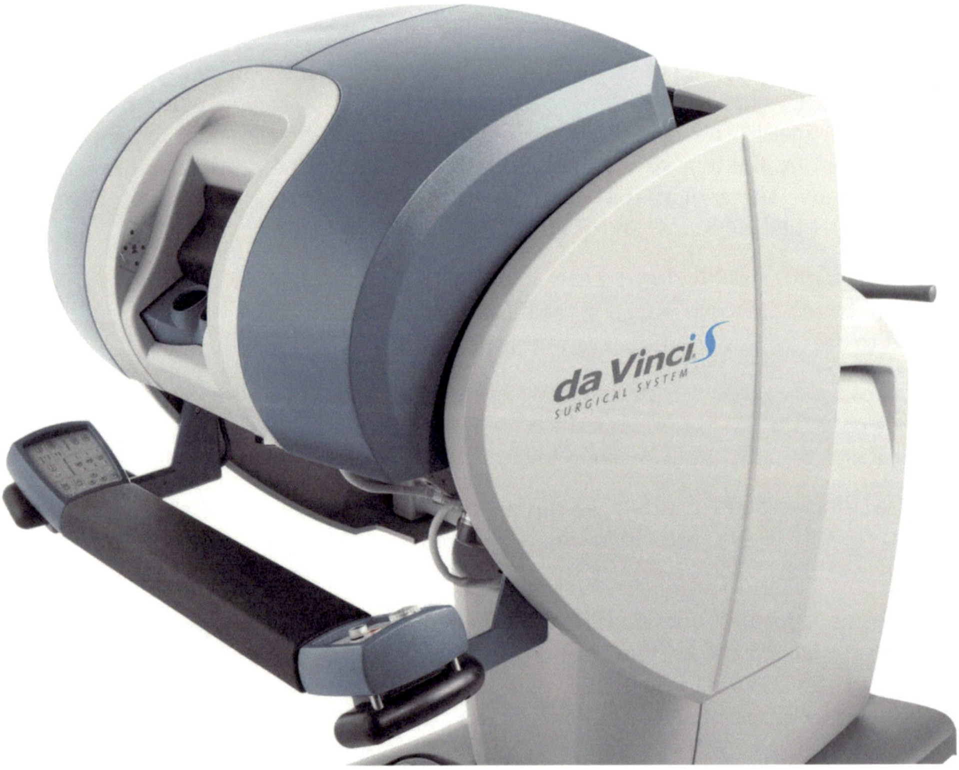


Fig. 1. "da Vinci S" surgeon's viewing and control console

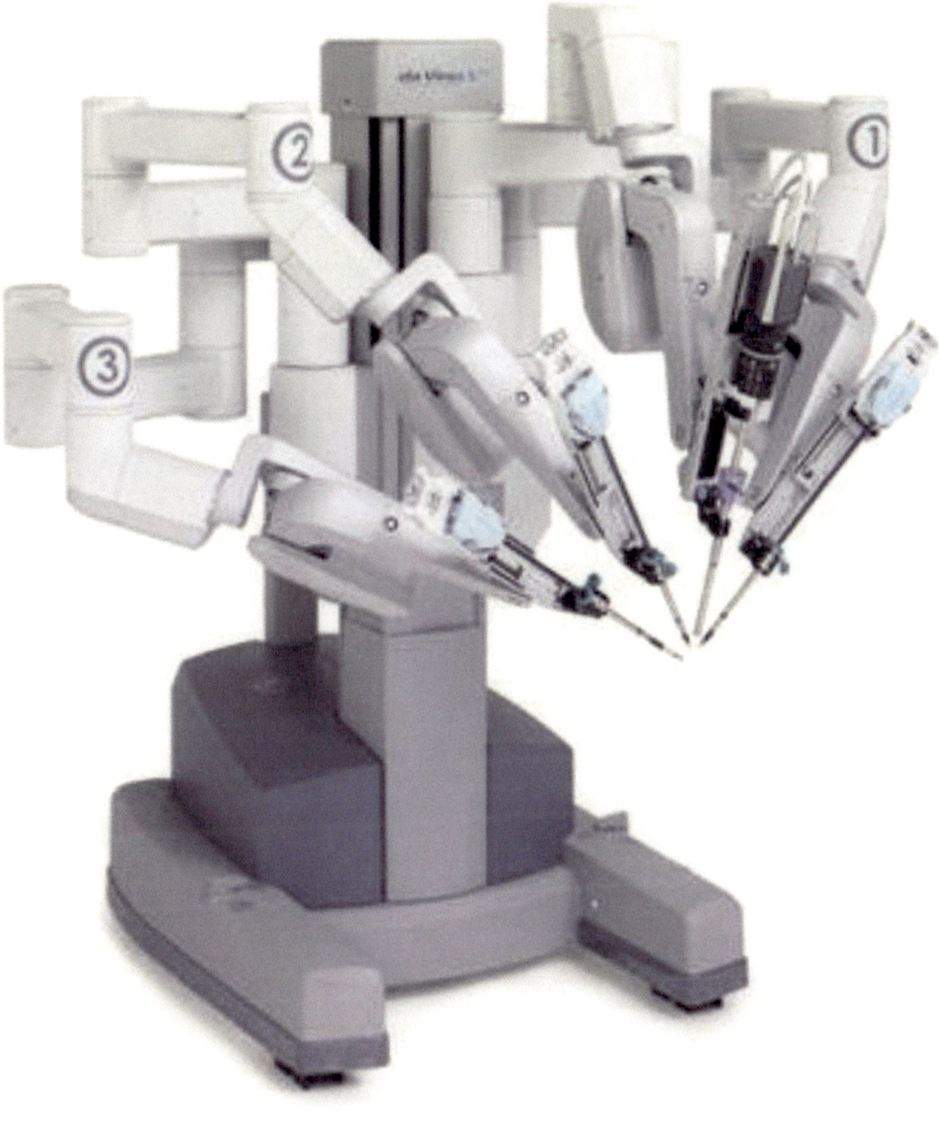


Fig. 2. "da Vinci S" robotic arms cart

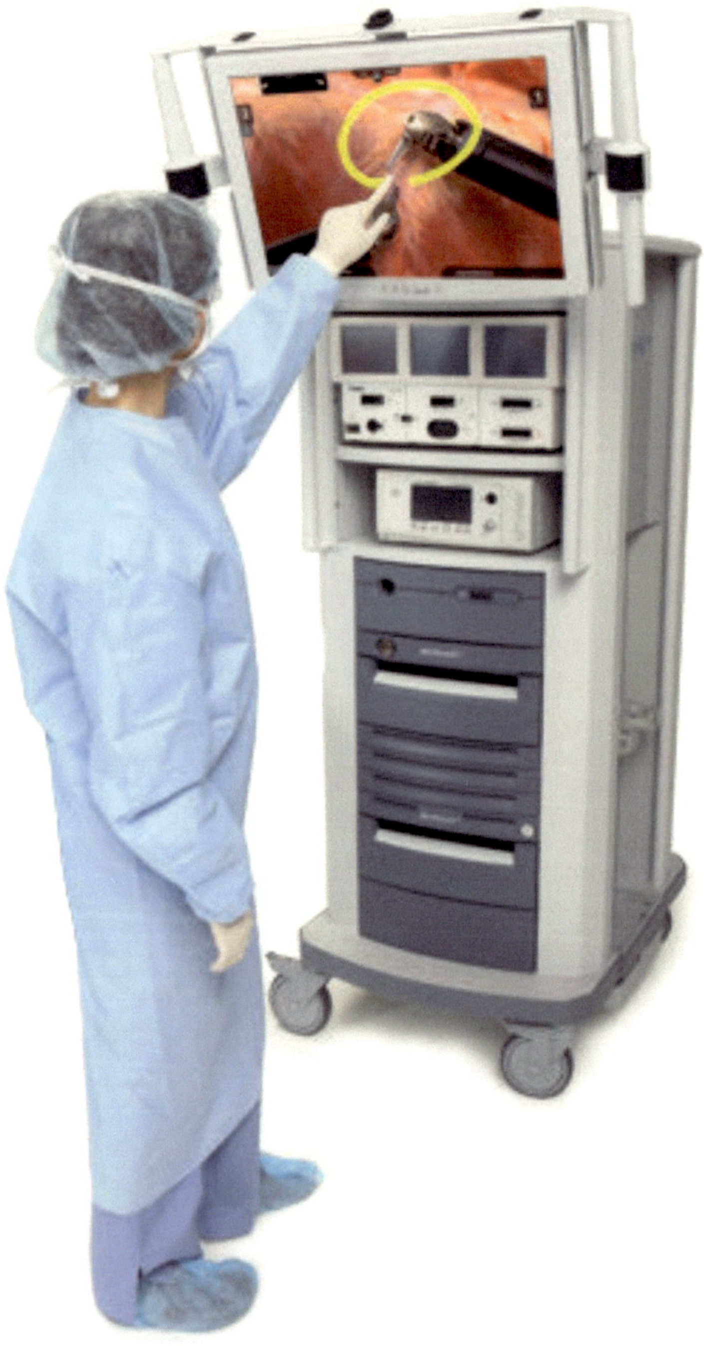

Fig. 3. The camera tower(the vision cart)

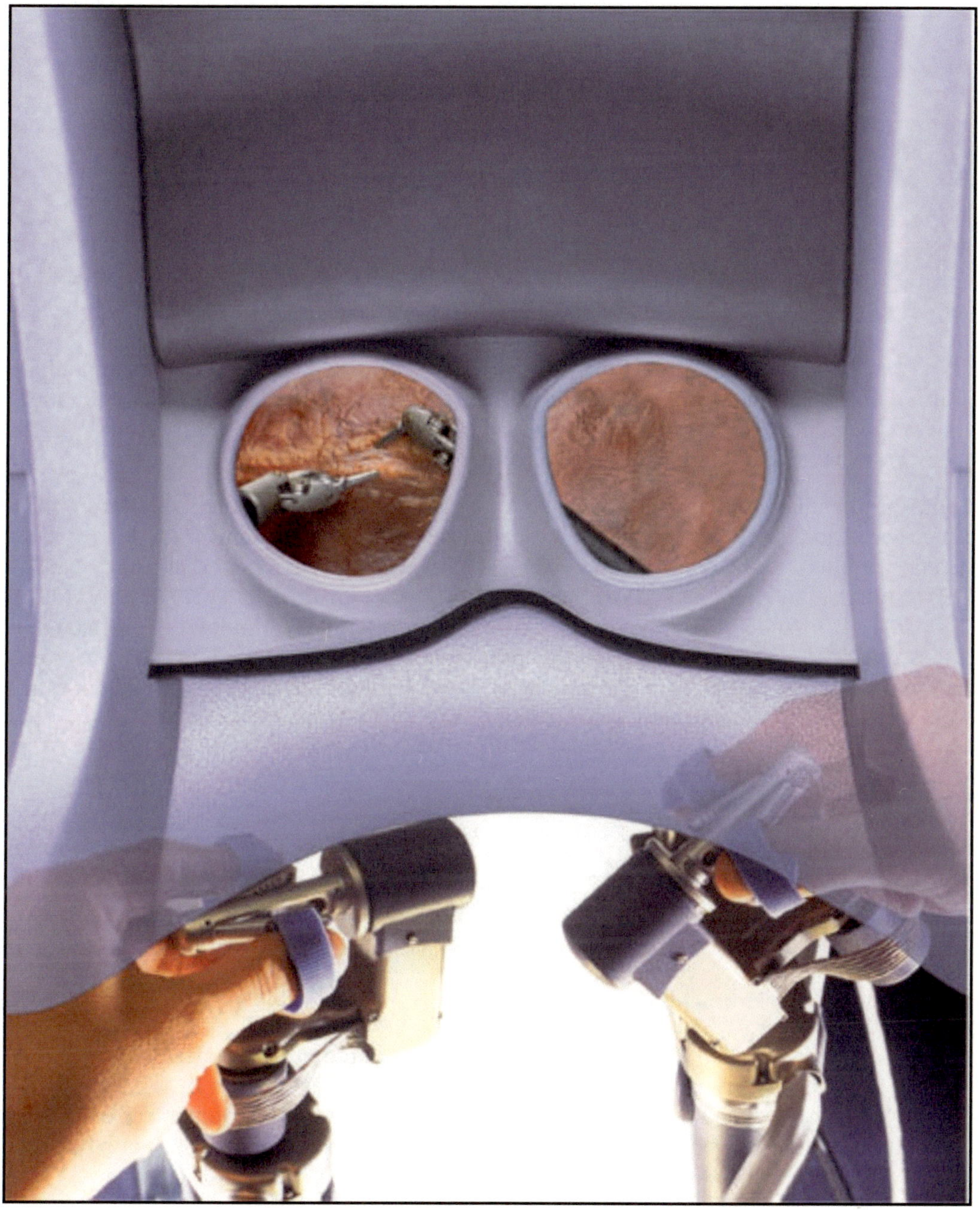

Fig. 4. The view through binoculars, a three-dimensional image

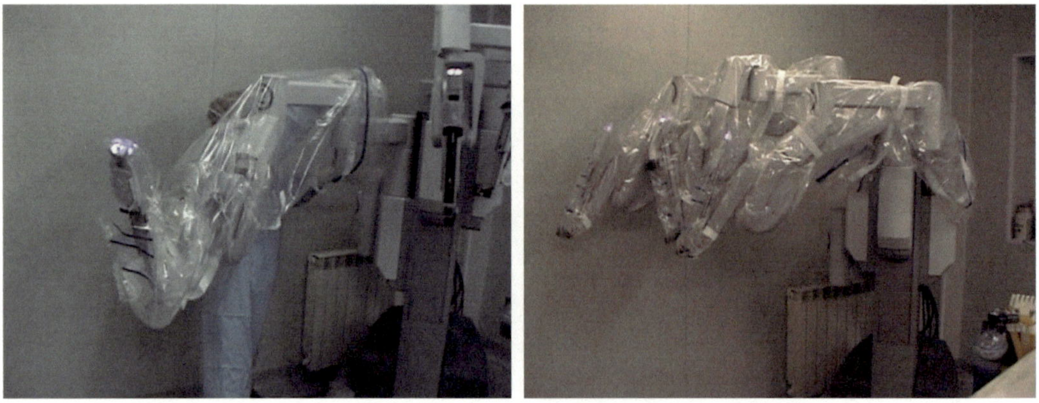

Fig. 5. Each instrument arm and the camera arm is draped separately

The vision cart contains controls for the cameras and light sources. It is a camera and a light source dedicated for each optical channel, for each of the surgeon's eyes. A $CO_2$ insufflations system can be mounted on this cart and also a monitor that allows the personnel in the operating room to view the intervention.

Some of the major advantages of robotic system are: stabile camera platform, three dimensional imaging, significant decrease limitation in the movement of instruments, tremor filtration and comfortable position for surgeon (Corcione et al. 2005, 19:117-119;Hashizume and Tsugawa 2004, 34:227-237;Ruckert et al. 2008, 1132:329-335;Tomulescu et al. 2009, 104:141-150). Another major advantage is offered by "Endowrist" instruments (fig 6) with 7 degrees of freedom - the arms have 3 degrees of freedom-pitch, yaw and insertion allow the appropriate instrument to move 2 additional degrees of freedom in the wrist and 2 additional motion for tool actuation.

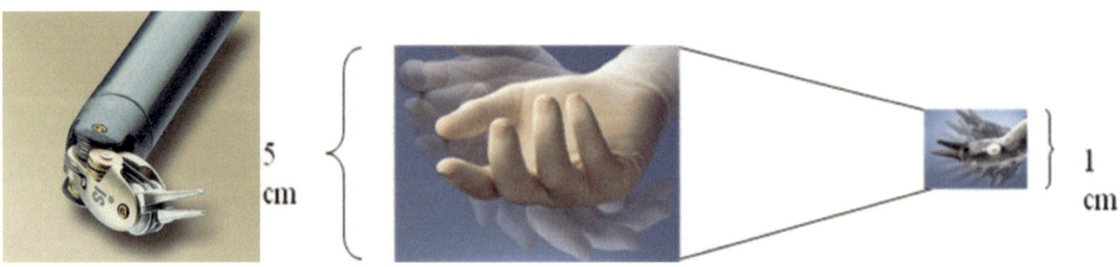


Fig. 6. Endo-wrist instruments

In 2001, Yoshino described the first robotic thymectomy in the treatment of small thymoma. In 2003, Ashton and Rea published a case report on robotic thymectomy in MG using two different approaches: the first adopted a right-sided approach with completion of the operation through a left-sided approach, the second used a left-sided approach only(Ashton, Jr. et al. 2003, 75:569-571;Rea et al. 2006, 81:455-459).

New opportunities for robots in general surgery are those interventions in which only the robot renders possible or noticeably simplifies a minimally invasive approach, i.e. procedures in which precise dissection of delicate, vulnerable anatomic structures take place in tiny areas with difficult access(Bodner et al. 2005, 135:674-678). Thymectomy is such a procedure and robotic surgery is the choice for extended minim invasive thymectomy. Based on a large experience (over 300 cases) with thoracoscopic thymectomy for nonthymomatous and thymomatous myasthenia gravis(Tomulescu et al. 2006, 82:1003-1007) we consider that the versatile instruments and better vision of robotic surgery permit us to make an extensive thymectomy easier and safer than in usual thoracoscopic approach despite the lack of tactile sense.

## 2. Operative technique

The operation is performed under general anesthesia. A double lumen endotracheal for selective single lung ventilation is used. As in classic thoracoscopic surgery use a right side or a left side approach is used in relation with surgeon preference. In fact the robot is only a better tool in performing the same unilateral extended thoracoscopic thymectomy robotic assisted.

For the left side approach the patient is positioned left side up 15-30$^{o}$ upon a bean bag. The left arm is positioned on a support, extended, axillary region well exposed. The video console is positioned at the head of the operating table. The robotic cart is on the right side of the patient 45$^{o}$ cranial (fig 7).

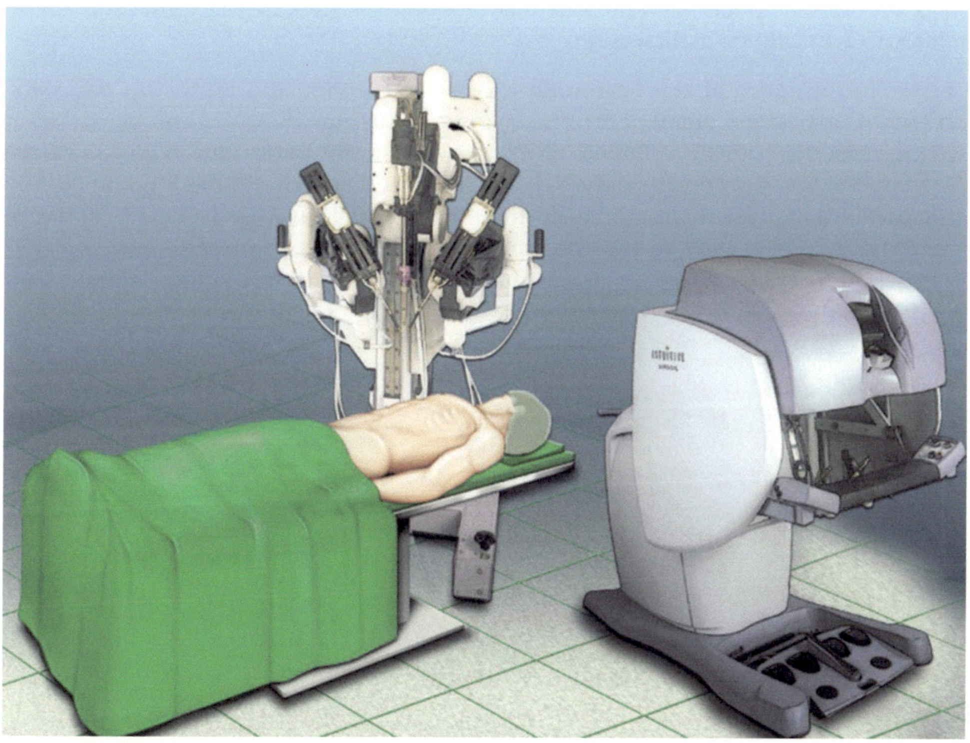

Fig. 7. Robotic carts positioning for thymectomy

The ports for the robotic arms are placed as follows: a camera port (12mm) in $5^{th}$ intercostals space on the anterior axillary line, and arm ports (8mm) in $5^{th}$ intercostals space on midclavicular line for left arm and in the $3^{rd}$ intercostals space on the anterior axillary line for the right arm. The arms of the robot are then attached to the trocar access points. The instruments are inserted under direct camera control. The left arm has an EndoWrist instrument for to grasp the thymus and in the right arm a dissection device that can be an Endo- Dissector, hook, scissor, or ultrasonic shears. One of the advantages of the robotic surgery is that we can change the instruments between the robotic arms and operate with the same dexterity with the left hand even if the surgeon is not ambidexterous. The ultrasonic shears has only 4 degrees of freedom and is not as maneuverable as EndoWrist instruments but can be used also for grasping and is not using monopolar electrocoagulation near the heart. I prefer to use a bipolar Micro-forceps for the left arm and a monopolar electrocoagulation scissor for the right arm. In this way we can use at maximum the excellent maneuverability of robotic instruments combining monopolar cautery dissection with bipolar coagulation using a very small forceps useful in the narrow space of the anterior mediastinum.

During surgery we inflate the thorax with $CO_2$, up to 10 mm Hg. The capnothorax facilitate the dissection, enlarge the space between sternum and pericardium, allowing us to have a better view contra laterally and in the cervical area. After a careful inspection we start the dissection at the left pericardiophrenic angle (in a left side approach).

We make an incision along the internal mammary artery and another along the phrenic nerve. We start in this way first of all to delimit the space of the thymus and fatty tissue that have to be excised in unilaterally extended robotic assisted thymectomy and secondly permit the $CO_2$ to help us in dissection.

We prefer to introduce at the beginning of the intervention the retrieving bag into the thorax. In this way every small part of fatty tissue or thymus dissected can be parked in it. Dissecting from the pericardiophrenic angle in the posterior pericardial plane and anterior retrosternal, the thymus and the fatty tissue is mobilized cranial, till the innominate vein is identified. The fatty tissue from the aortopulmonary window is dissected in the same manner. The excellent view of the robotic system allows us to identify and protégé the phrenic nerve, recurrent nerve and vagus. The dissection continue contra laterally, on the right side with the dissection of the inferior thymus horn.

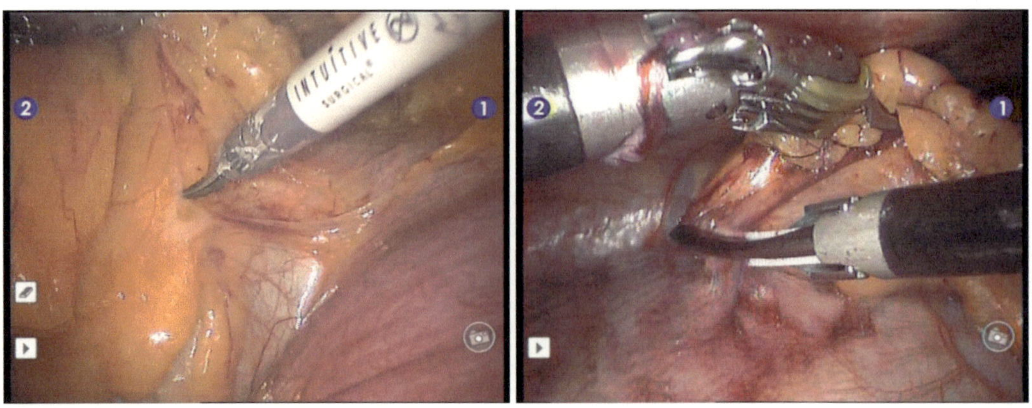


Fig. 8. Starting the operation at the pericardiophrenic angle

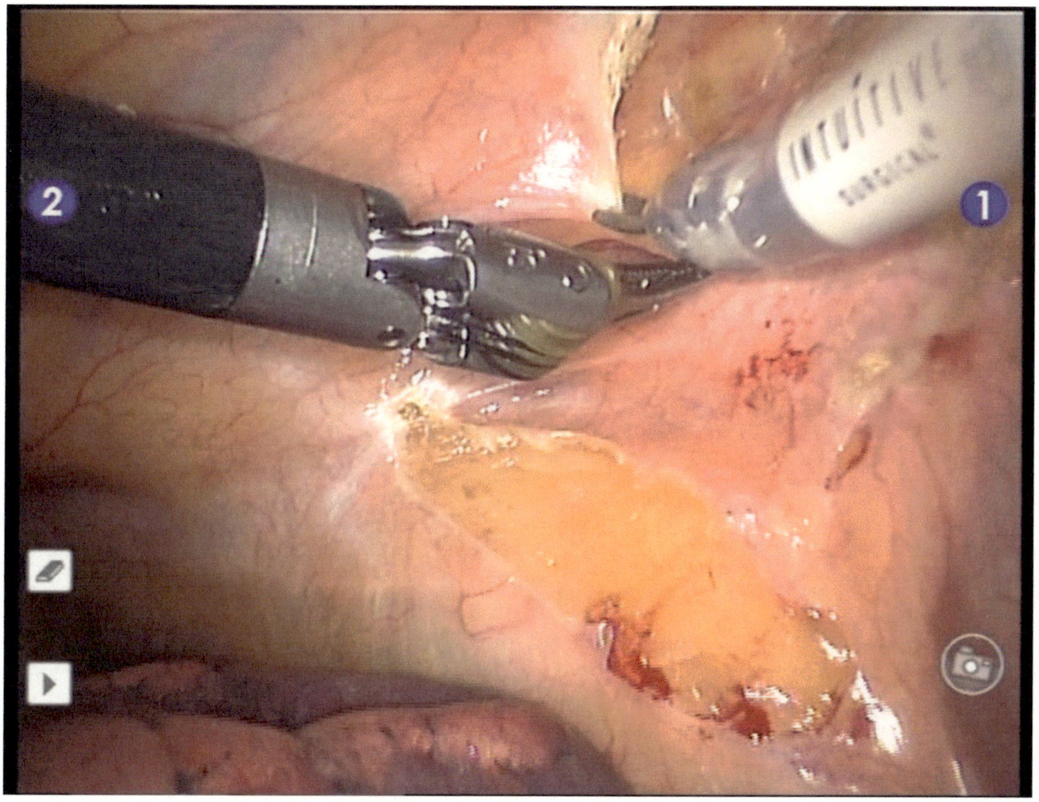


Fig. 9. Delimit the operation field (right side approach)

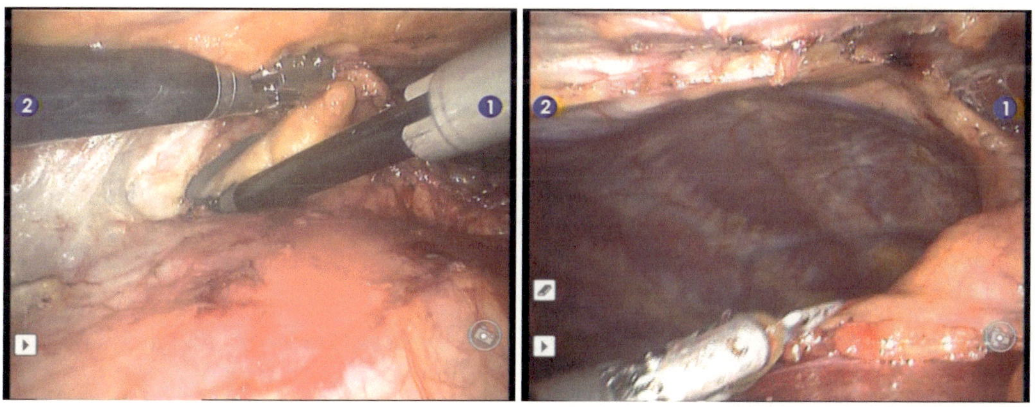


Fig. 10. Dissection continues contra-laterally (left side approach)

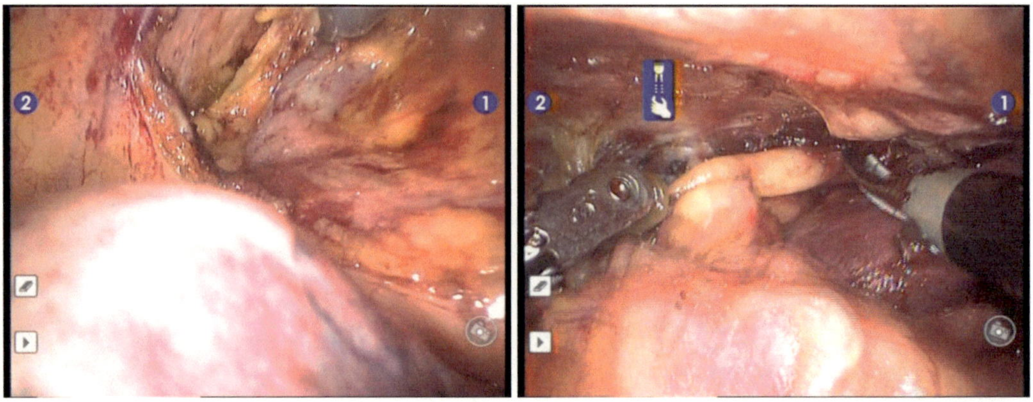

Fig. 11. Dissection of the upper horns from inominate vein (a right side approach, b left side approach)

At the superior level the thymus and the fatty tissue is dissected along the border of the inominate vein indentifying the thymic veins, clipping and sectioning them. The dissection continues in the cervical area with the dissection of the upper thymus horns (fig 9). Sectioning the upper horns vessels coming from the cervical area permit us to mobilize the upper horns caudally by applying gentle traction. There is an detail to be noticed, robotic system does not have force feed-back so there is no tactile sense. A surgeon have to teach himself to feel with the eyes when is performing robotic surgery.

At the end all thymus and fatty tissue in the anterior mediastinum from diaphragm to the cervical area is excised performing a unilaterally extended robotic assisted thymectomy. The specimen placed in the retrieval bag and removed by an enlarged trocar incision. Drainage finalizes the intervention. We have presented a left side approach, the right side is performed in the same way, the decision to use a right or a left side approach being in relation to surgeon point of view and experience and previous patient interventions.

## 3. Our results

In 2008 a „da Vinci S" robotic system was acquired in the "Dan Setlacec" Center of General Surgery and Liver Transplantation of Fundeni Clinical Institute. Till now we have performed a unilaterally extended robotic assisted thymectomy in 40 cases. The study population consisted of 11 males (27.5%) and 29 females (72.5%) with an median age of 36.25 years (range 11- 67 years)

A left thoracoscopic approach was used for 35 of the patients (87.5%) and a right thoracoscopic approach for 5 of the patients (12.5%). Decision to use the right-side or left-side approach was considered in relation with the CT aspect of each patient's thymus. There were no conversions to open thymectomy.

The mean operative time was of 115+/-40 min. There was zero mortality and morbidity was observed in 1 patient (2.5%) with contralateral pneumothorax after drain removal.

The following histological diagnoses were made: normal thymus in 5 patients (12.5%), involuted thymus in 9 patients (22.5%) and thymus hypertrophy (hyperplastic thymus) in 26 patients (65%). The average weight of the thymus was 100 g (range: 75-150 g).

The mean length of hospitalization was 3.25 days (range: 2-5 days)

## 4. Conclusions

Robotic surgery has affirmed itself as an evolution of minimal invasive approach allowing surgeons to overcome some limitations of classic thoracoscopy. Robotically is possible to perform an extended unilaterally thymectomy in a more complete and safe way despite the lack of tactile sense with results superior to thoracoscopic thymectomy(Ruckert, Swierzy, and Ismail 2011, 141:673-677). Even a major hemorrhagic incident as clip dislocation on thymus vein can be solved by suturing with 6O Prolene. (fig12). The versatile robotic instruments allowed performing suture at an angle that would have not been possible using a thoracoscopic approach.

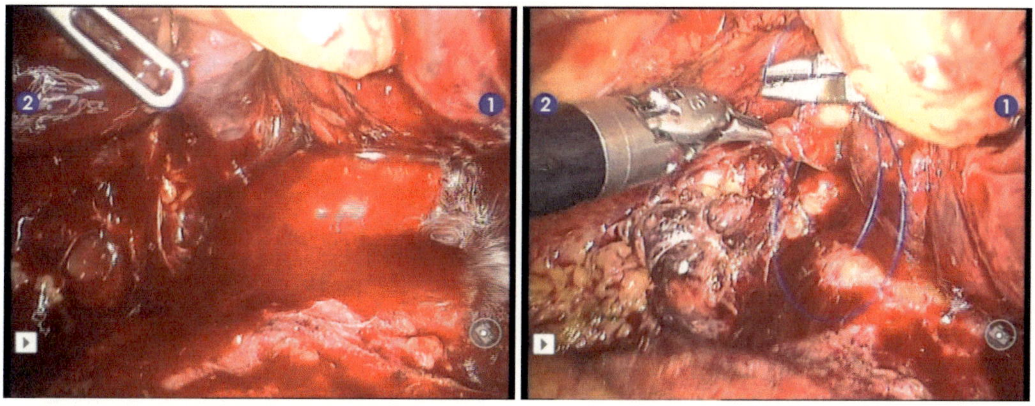


Fig. 12. Suture of the thymus vein disruption

We have also to be aware that there are also some limitations that came with the robotic system. During the procedure is difficult to place additional ports and to change the position of the operating table. The camera can be placed only in a 12 mm port and this can be difficult in children. Due to the variable distance between the console surgeon and the patient we consider the importance of side assistant surgeon(s) vital for an uneventful surgical procedure. They should be well trained surgeons in general surgery, advanced laparoscopic procedures and robotics. There is a need for improvement for ultrasonic shears in order to have the same versatility as the Endowrist instruments. The lack of tactile sense could be a challenge for beginners. In spite the need of these improvements we can conclude that the system is still underused regarding its possibilities.

Because the movements in robotic surgery are intuitive and the visualization is superior to traditional surgical techniques, proctoring and training in this advanced minimally invasive procedure is more rapid and efficient than with a classic thoracoscopic approach or transcervical thymectomy(Calhoun et al. 1999, 230:555-559;Shrager 2010, 89:S2128-S2134).

We encountered no brachial plexus injury, as was reported by Mong-Wei Lin and co-workers(Lin et al. 2010, 37:7-12) and Ravindra Pandey and co-workers(Pandey et al. 2009, 23:584-586) using a robotic approach, but we have taken extreme care regarding patient positioning, avoiding 90° abduction in the placement of the shoulder joint and placing a roll under the arm and axilla in these patients. The anaesthesiologist and the assistant surgeon were constantly looking for any injury that the robotic arms could potentially cause. Continuous communication between the console surgeon and the other two members of the surgical-anaesthesiology team and careful procedure planning are the keys of good results with robotic surgery.

## 5. References


Ashton RC, Jr., McGinnis KM, Connery CP, Swistel DG, Ewing DR, and Derose JJ, Jr. 2003. Totally endoscopic robotic thymectomy for myasthenia gravis. *Ann. Thorac. Surg.* 75 (2): 569-571.

Bodner J, Augustin F, Wykypiel H, Fish J, Muehlmann G, Wetscher G, and Schmid T. 2005. The da Vinci robotic system for general surgical applications: a critical interim appraisal. *Swiss. Med. Wkly.* 135 (45-46): 674-678.

Calhoun RF, Ritter JH, Guthrie TJ, Pestronk A, Meyers BF, Patterson GA, Pohl MS, and Cooper JD. 1999. Results of transcervical thymectomy for myasthenia gravis in 100 consecutive patients. *Ann. Surg.* 230 (4): 555-559.

Corcione F, Esposito C, Cuccurullo D, Settembre A, Miranda N, Amato F, Pirozzi F, and Caiazzo P. 2005. Advantages and limits of robot-assisted laparoscopic surgery: preliminary experience. *Surg. Endosc.* 19 (1): 117-119.

Hashizume M, and Tsugawa K. 2004. Robotic surgery and cancer: the present state, problems and future vision. *Jpn. J. Clin. Oncol.* 34 (5): 227-237.

Lin MW, Chang YL, Huang PM, and Lee YC. 2010. Thymectomy for non-thymomatous myasthenia gravis: a comparison of surgical methods and analysis of prognostic factors. *Eur. J. Cardiothorac. Surg.* 37 (1): 7-12.

Pandey R, Elakkumanan LB, Garg R, Jyoti B, Mukund C, Chandralekha, Punj J, and Vanlal D. 2009. Brachial plexus injury after robotic-assisted thoracoscopic thymectomy. *J. Cardiothorac. Vasc. Anesth.* 23 (4): 584-586.

Rea F, Marulli G, Bortolotti L, Feltracco P, Zuin A, and Sartori F. 2006. Experience with the "da Vinci" robotic system for thymectomy in patients with myasthenia gravis: report of 33 cases. *Ann. Thorac. Surg.* 81 (2): 455-459.

Ruckert JC, Ismail M, Swierzy M, Sobel H, Rogalla P, Meisel A, Wernecke KD, Ruckert RI, and Muller JM. 2008. Thoracoscopic thymectomy with the da Vinci robotic system for myasthenia gravis. *Ann. N. Y. Acad. Sci.* 1132: 329-335.

Ruckert JC, Swierzy M, and Ismail M. 2011. Comparison of robotic and nonrobotic thoracoscopic thymectomy: a cohort study. *J. Thorac. Cardiovasc. Surg.* 141 (3): 673-677.

Shrager JB. 2010. Extended transcervical thymectomy: the ultimate minimally invasive approach. *Ann. Thorac. Surg.* 89 (6): S2128-S2134.

Tomulescu V, Ion V, Kosa A, Sgarbura O, and Popescu I. 2006. Thoracoscopic thymectomy mid-term results. *Ann. Thorac. Surg.* 82 (3): 1003-1007.

Tomulescu V, Stanciulea O, Balescu I, Vasile S, Tudor S, Gheorghe C, Vasilescu C, and Popescu I. 2009. First year experience of robotic-assisted laparoscopic surgery with 153 cases in a general surgery department: indications, technique and results. *Chirurgia. (Bucur. )* 104 (2): 141-150.

Vasilescu C, and Popescu I. 2008. Chirurgia robotica - problemele inceputului; posbilitati si perspective. *Chirurgia. (Bucur. )* 103 (1): 9-11.